INTERVIEWING FOR QUALITATIVE INQUIRY

Also from Ruthellen Josselson

Five Ways of Doing Qualitative Analysis:
Phenomenological Psychology, Grounded Theory, Discourse
Analysis, Narrative Research, and Intuitive Inquiry
Frederick J. Wertz, Kathy Charmaz, Linda M. McMullen,
Ruthellen Josselson, Rosemarie Anderson, and Emalinda McSpadden

Interviewing for Qualitative Inquiry

A Relational Approach

RUTHELLEN JOSSELSON

THE GUILFORD PRESS
New York   London

© 2013 The Guilford Press
A Division of Guilford Publications, Inc.
72 Spring Street, New York, NY 10012
www.guilford.com

Printed in the United States of America

This book is printed on acid-free paper.

Last digit is print number: 9   8   7   6   5   4   3   2   1

The author has checked with sources believed to be reliable in her efforts to provide information that is complete and generally in accord with the standards of practice that are accepted at the time of publication. However, in view of the possibility of human error or changes in behavioral, mental health, or medical sciences, neither the author, nor the editor and publisher, nor any other party who has been involved in the preparation or publication of this work warrants that the information contained herein is in every respect accurate or complete, and they are not responsible for any errors or omissions or the results obtained from the use of such information. Readers are encouraged to confirm the information contained in this book with other sources.

Library of Congress Cataloging-in-Publication Data

Josselson, Ruthellen.
    Interviewing for qualitative inquiry : a relational approach /
Ruthellen Josselson. — first edition.
        pages   cm
    Includes bibliographical references and index.
    ISBN 978-1-4625-1000-9 (pbk. : alk. paper) — ISBN 978-1-4625-1004-7
(hardcover : alk. paper)
    1. Interviewing.   I. Title.
    BF637.I5J67 2013
    001.4′33—dc23

                                                              2013001286

I hear things people badly want to tell, but don't tell because they are afraid no one can understand.

—ROBERTSON DAVIES, *The Manticore*

ACKNOWLEDGMENTS

I wish to thank a number of people who have contributed their ideas to this book. First of all, I thank Amia Lieblich, my collaborator in every aspect of qualitative inquiry, who has been my inspiration, my sounding board, and my supporter for more than 20 years. Hanoch Flum, my husband, himself a qualitative researcher, assisted me in many ways, offering his ideas and experiences and his close reading. He also put me in touch with some of his students, whom I thank for their useful contributions. I also thank Beverly Palmer and Marilyn Freimuth, who have contributed ideas to improve this book. I am grateful to many students from Europe, Israel, and the United States who have participated in my workshops and taught me about dilemmas of interviewing that I would not have discovered on my own. Two of my students at the Fielding Graduate University, Heidi Mattila and Jeanne Miller, read an earlier draft of this book and advised me about how students might use it to learn. I am grateful to Sharon Kangisser Cohen, who not only allowed but encouraged me to use the "difficult" interview she conducted. I am indebted to all of those who have been participants in my research, who, through their efforts to help me learn about their lives in relation to my research questions, have taught me how to interview better. They, of course, will always remain anonymous. I also thank my editor at The Guilford Press, C. Deborah Laughton, for her enthusiasm and support of this project, and Marie Sprayberry for her very thoughtful and careful copyediting. Finally, I am grateful to the reviewers, whose criticism was highly constructive: Elizabeth Monk-Turner (Department of Sociology and Criminal Justice, Old Dominion University); Penny Burge (School of Education, Virginia Tech); Carey Andrzejewski (College of Education, Auburn University); and Terrie Vann-Ward (School of Nursing, University of Utah). I am also grateful to the people who gave me permission to use excerpts from their interviews in this book.

PRCE

The next necessary thing . . . is to enlarge the possibility
of an intelligible discourse between people quite different
from one another in interest, outlook, wealth, and power,
and yet contained in a world where, tumbled as they are
into endless connection, it is increasingly difficult to get
out of each other's way.

— CLIFFORD GEERTZ

This book is for people whose research questions lead them to conduct in-depth research interviews in order to obtain data that will help them better understand the *processes* of the phenomena of interest to them. This mode of inquiry may be categorized as "qualitative" or "narrative" research[1]; it is utilized when research questions concern how people understand and make meaning of facets of their lives. The light beam of investigation is generally pointed either at the internal world—how people (perhaps of a particular subgroup) make inner meaning out of particular experiences—or at the external world—how particular social institutions or cultural phenomena are experienced by people. Sometimes researchers are trying to do both, as in reading the culture from individual experiences and understanding how cultural experience creates or shapes the self. In either case, the investigation will focus

---

[1] In this book, I use the terms "narrative" and "qualitative" interchangeably, although I recognize that qualitative research encompasses more than the narrative approach, including focus groups, participant observation, and action research. The kind of interviewing I detail is aimed at eliciting narratives of lived experience in a two-person setting.

on experience and meanings—how people going about their lives have interpreted or made personal sense out of some event, developmental change, or social phenomenon. The researcher in such an investigation is interested in plumbing the depths and complexities of some issue, trying to enlarge rather than reduce the picture already present in the scholarly literature. To do that, the researcher is trying to understand the research participant holistically, as an experiencing, meaning-making person. This necessitates large segments of talk that reflect the participant's subjective ways of being in the world; the research is aimed at gathering experiential accounts in the participants' own words. Whether the analytic method will be grounded theory, narrative analysis, phenomenological analysis, discourse analysis, or any other approach, a good interview is necessary to create the data that will be used to explore the research question.[2]

In research projects that call for this form of interviewing as data collection, the interest is in people as actors rather than as witnesses. The intent is to understand how people construct or interpret their experiences, rather than piecing together views of an external event. For example, in the wake of some natural disaster, news media might be interested in reconstructing an account of what happened and might interview witnesses about what they saw or heard; a research project looking at the effects of disaster would be aimed at how what people saw or heard affected their lives after the tragedy—how they coped with shock, trauma, memories, or loss. Therefore, this book focuses on how to interview a participant in order to obtain a view of the participant's internal world (which will, of course, include representations of the external world as the participant experienced it).

The purpose of studying other people in depth is not to measure, predict, or classify them. Our purpose is to *understand*, more extensively or more deeply, other people's experiences of some aspect of their lives. Our focus is on subjectivity.

---

[2]An excellent introduction to analytic approaches is Wertz et al. (2011), which presents five different ways of analyzing the same interview. See also Lieblich, Tuval-Mashiach, and Zilber (1998) and Creswell (2012).

While a prestructured list of questions to be asked may be appropriate for survey-research kinds of investigations, narrative research requires interview techniques that will enable the disclosure of multilayered individual meanings. Sometimes called "depth interviewing," the form of interview to be considered here aims for a rich, nuanced, *storied* sample of subjectivity that details how it has felt to the participant to be living the life he or she has lived in relation to the phenomena of the research question. Later, after the interview, the researcher will transcribe the recordings to text, and then will spend hours poring over the texts to find themes or patterns and to make interpretations of the text that might shed light on the initial research question.

There is already an enormous literature on interviewing and the epistemological ground on which its assumptions stand. Questions about what it means to ask another person to narrate his or her experiences have engaged scholars because they reflect profound issues about the nature of reality, the social construction of meanings, and what it means to know (Roulston, 2010). In this book, I assume that readers are familiar with some of this scholarship.[3] Most books on interviewing have extensive material about conceptualizing the interviewing process, but little on conducting the interview itself. The reader may learn a great deal about how to *think* about the interview and its place in research, but little about how actually to conduct it. I have been astonished at how many books that purport to explain the method of interviewing do not go beyond suggesting that the interviewer pose open-ended questions and establish rapport. Both "open-ended questions" and "rapport," however, are complex processes that require elaboration and detailing. In nearly all texts on interviewing, qualitative researchers are implored to listen carefully and respectfully, and to make interpretations of transcribed texts meticulously and judiciously, attending to the nuances of how the conversation unfolds.[4] Yet there are few guidelines to

---

[3]See Bruner (1990), Kvale and Brinkmann (2009), MacIntyre (2007), Polkinghorne (1988), Sarbin (1986), and Wertz et al. (2011).

[4]See, for example, Alvesson and Skoldberg (2009), Atkinson, Coffey, Delamont,

what it means to listen carefully and respectfully, or how actually to respond in the interview space.

Whatever the researcher finally does with interview texts, interpretation is limited by the nature and quality of the interview itself. What the interviewee can and does narrate depends on what is happening in the actual interview situation and is wholly influenced by the dynamics of the *research relationship*. Interviewing, in this view, is not a procedure, but an interpersonal process—one that can be analyzed and understood. My goal here is to focus on the relational dynamics of the interview from an intersubjective perspective.

Listening is an active process, but the activity of listening is not apparent. One can describe how to ask questions, because questions are verbal and visible. Listening, though, is internal. Nevertheless, interviewees can "feel" when another person is fully listening. When people feel "heard" as the result of good listening, they are inclined to tell more, to struggle to find words for experiences that aren't easily described, or even to tell about reactions and meanings that they have never before put in words or felt comfortable telling to anyone. As a psychologist, my main research interest is in detailing the internal world, reaching emotional and meaning-making levels of human experience to understand the psychological processes that underlie how people go about their lives. My approach to interviewing, however, is also suitable for those who have more sociological interests and would like to understand social institutions or subcultures as the people who constitute these institutions or subcultures experience them.

The narrative interview is a special kind of conversation where general guidelines of exploration can be offered, but once the interactional, intersubjective journey begins, few firm rules can be applied. In other forms of research, there are instruments and procedures. In interview-based research, the interviewer is the instrument and the procedure. Therefore, it is extremely important to understand as fully as possible one's own contribution, as the interviewer,

---

Lofland, and Lofland (2001), Gubrium and Holstein (2002), Kvale (1996), Seidman (2006), and Weiss (1994), which all set out these principles.

to the co-construction of experience that the interview represents. The richness and value of an interview depend on the relational and empathic skills of the interviewer. Interviewing is an art, but it is an art that can be learned, and one's skill with it can be increased.

The story is perhaps apocryphal, but I have heard that Henri Matisse told his art students to go see a flower for the first time. This is much like what we do in a narrative research interview. We may know a great deal about the topic, but the person before us is brand-new. There are two potential errors we can make. If we structure the interview plan too much, we restrict what we can see; we are likely to learn "facts" but not meanings, and little about the uniqueness of our participant (we may discover only that flowers have petals and stems). If we provide too little structure, the participant may talk, but not about what we are interested in (we want to see a flower, not a car). We must provide "just enough" structure so that we learn something new that relates to our question. We want to encounter the uniqueness of *this* flower in its "flowerness," so that we may better understand and illuminate something about this kind of flower that we didn't see before. Qualitative research is about discovery of something new.

A narrative interview is open-ended and extended. It is focused initially on a topic of interest to the researcher, but interviewees are encouraged to place their own meanings into the dialogue. The nuances of experience, the subtleties of subjectivity, and the shadings of thought and emotion are the focus of attention.

Over the past 20 years, I have been doing workshops in the United States and abroad to teach people in psychology, sociology, anthropology, education, nursing, gerontology, oral history, and social work how to conduct interviews for research purposes. This book is an effort to write down what my students have most wanted to know, and to respond to the questions they most frequently raise. I think that all too often, graduate programs allow students to do interview-based research without proper training, as though interviewing is a skill that is somehow innate and students just know how to do it. After all, isn't it just asking people questions? No, it is not. And I strongly counsel supervision and collaboration groups as necessary for developing the skill to conduct narrative interviews. I have written this book as a guide that might be used in a qualitative research course of study, but it could also be used by small groups of students working together to do the practice exercises. My aim here is both to teach new interviewers basic skills and to help more experienced people enhance their repertoire of interventions.

I have written this book as a hands-on guide for practice. I offer "tips" and specific instructions, and often take the liberty of addressing you, the reader, directly, because, in my mind, I am having a conversation with you, often imagining your response to what I say. I think of interviewing as a special kind of conversation, and I think of this book as yet another kind of conversation.

I have been doing interview-based research for over 40 years, and with each project and each participant, I learn more about the nuances of managing this very particular human encounter. My overall aim is to try to pass forward to the next generation of qualitative researchers what I have learned.

Plan of the Book

The process and content of the interview are intertwined. In this book, I often shift focus from one to the other. Because they interpenetrate, this cannot be done in a linear way—so I ask you, the reader, to bear with me if I seem to circle back and forth at times.

Chapter 1, "The Foundations of Interviewing as Qualitative Inquiry," briefly sets out the epistemological grounding for qualitative research interviews, recognizing that they are situated in very particular contexts. I develop the idea that human experience is *storied* and that the aim of the narrative interview is to invite the telling of storied accounts. The content of what is told reflects the process of the telling. The depth and meanings of what a participant discloses in an interview depend on the nature of the research relationship— which is a major focus throughout the book.

In Chapter 2, "Introduction to the Research Relationship," I examine in detail the formation of the research relationship from the inception of the research project through recruitment of participants and the first moments of meeting. An ethical attitude to the process is essential, as is attunement to the myriad feelings the interview situation arouses in both the interviewer and the interviewee. I consider the intricate dynamics of what takes place when one person is "observing" or "seeing" the other.

Chapter 3, "Planning the Interview," turns to issues of structure in considering the design of the interview in relation to the conceptual question of the research. It outlines the distinction between the organizing research question and the experience-near question that is designed to engage narration of the participant's experiences. I give examples of moving from the conceptual question to the recruitment question to the question that orients the interview itself. This chapter also considers the issues involved in mapping the range of questions to be explored in the interview.

Turning back to a focus on the process of the interview, Chapter 4, "Beginning the Interview," first discusses the mechanics of meeting; it then shifts to how the interviewer presents him- or herself to the interviewee and what issues are likely to arise at the start of an interview. This chapter discusses the first moves in the interview dance as the research relationship gets under way. I offer detailed pointers about how to position oneself and one's verbal responses in order to foster an open, exploratory, rich, and detailed sharing of the participant's experience. The chapter also discusses, with examples, the primary response stances within an active listening framework, including silence, clarification, confrontation, and empathic response. The aim is to move with the participant to create an attentive, nonjudgmental, empathic arena for the interview conversation.

Chapter 5, "The Empathic Attitude of Listening," further describes the use of empathy in the service of obtaining richly detailed interviews. The interviewer must track both feeling and the cognitive aspects of experience in order to try to understand the experience from the participant's point of view. By summarizing, paraphrasing, or mirroring, the interviewer expresses empathic contact, and this encourages deeper and more extensive elaboration of the participant's experience. This chapter offers dialogues that illustrate examples of the kinds of choices the interviewer makes in groping for accurate empathy.

In Chapter 6, "The Research Relationship, Part II: Ethics and Humanity," I return to issues of process in the research relationship. Interviewing in qualitative research invokes an often intimate connection between the researcher and the participant, and the researcher is treading on unfamiliar and emotionally charged relational ground. I offer guidelines about how the researcher can both be fully human and also stay in the researcher role. Issues of ethics are pervasive in this relationship, and I distinguish an ethical human research relationship from the formalities of ethical practice.

Chapter 7, "The Good Interview," presents three very different examples of what I consider to be good interviews, each with particular challenges. I demonstrate how the empathic stance elicits elaborated, meaningful narratives that are layered and complex. In Chapter 8, "Learning from Bad and Difficult Interviews," I list and illustrate common mistakes of novice interviewers, and I discuss some "difficult" types of interviewees that researchers may encounter. I also present a very challenging interview and discuss how the challenges were met.

In Chapter 9, "Dos and Don'ts of Interviewing," I offer some brief, illustrated "pointers" for researchers to keep in mind while interviewing. Chapter 10, "After the Interview," comments on transcription, takes up the issue of member checking, and discusses the research relationship following the interview, especially issues of writing about the participants. I stress the importance of the research relationship even at the analysis stage.

CONTENTS

Contents

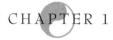

CHAPTER 1

The Foundations
of Interviewing
as Qualitative Inquiry

Epistemological Grounding

An interview is a shared product of *what* two people—one the interviewer, the other the interviewee—talk about and *how* they talk together. Some meeting of two minds occurs through this conversation. There is no longer much scholarly doubt that what is in the mind of the interviewer influences the process and content of "the data." There is, however, much scholarly debate about how to think about the co-construction of the interview. If there is no "objective" account to be unearthed in the interview, then what can we learn from talking to others about their experiences? And if we re-present accounts of experience that our interviewees tell us about, are we somehow falling into unreflexive realist assumptions?

Most interview-based qualitative research is located somewhere between realist and relativistic approaches to knowledge (Denzin & Lincoln, 2011; Roulston, 2010). That is, we qualitative researchers recognize that reality is socially constructed and that we have a part in creating, through our framing of questions and our forms

1

of investigation and analysis, the very phenomena we study (Gergen, 2009). We also understand that people construct their own social reality (Berger & Luckmann, 1966; Gergen, 1994). We are aware that we as researchers are the authors of our interpretations; yet we aim, through interviewing, to learn something about what is beyond ourselves and our preexisting assumptions.

To base a research project on interviews is to assume that there is some knowable reality beyond our own minds. While I acknowledge the need for a careful, ongoing, critical scrutiny of the interpretive process at every stage of the research, I focus more closely in this book on the process of creating the data through carefully crafted interviews. I consider the ways in which the interview itself is a form of evolving constructed interpretation. Yet I am writing from the position (shared, I think, by most qualitative inquirers) that although reality is co-constructed, we can reach some understanding of others' experiences of their lives. As Sayer (1992) points out, although human phenomena cannot exist independently of social forces, they usually have some independence from the particular people who are studying them.

Our ultimate interpretive role as researchers is to understand people better—or at least differently—than they understand themselves. The aim of interviewing is to document people's experience, self-understanding, and working models of the world they live in, so that we may later attempt to make meaning of these phenomena at levels of analysis beyond simple descriptions of what we heard.

Most qualitative investigations ground themselves in "hermeneutics," the science of meaning making—an approach to knowledge production that involves reading a text so that layers of intention and meaning can be understood.[1] As scholars, our aim is to begin with the phenomenology of experience, and then to try to puzzle out the dynamics and structures that may account for that experience. However we conceive our plan for doing so, we must begin with good data of experience, which we can only obtain from a well-conducted interview.

The kinds of data that are created with in-depth qualitative

---

[1]See Josselson (2004) and Messer, Sass, and Woolfolk (1988).

interviewing reflect narrative truth rather than historical truth (Spence, 1984). Interview data do not create a picture of some (unknowable) objective reality. Rather, they allow us to encounter the mental sets of the interviewee—the subjectively created reality in which the interviewee experiences life (Fosshage, 1995). Our aim is to obtain a broad and rich picture of this reality, which will inevitably depict the schemas or constructions through which the participant engages the world. As researchers, we pay attention to both the content of the narration (the *told*) and the structure of the narration (the *telling*). The phrasing used by participants and the particular words they choose indicate something about how they locate themselves (or find themselves positioned) in the social world.

Meaning and Interpretation: The Role of Stories

Meaning making and interpretation are at the center of narrative research projects. The aim is to build a layered, complex understanding of some aspect of human experience, in which linkages between themes are of interest to a researcher. The data of interest are people's stories of life experience, rather than their decontextualized opinions, attitudes, or facts about life.

Human life is composed of stories. Narratives construct memory, organize time, and create identity (Ricoeur, 1981; MacIntyre, 2007); stories integrate facts and feelings (Fulford, 1999). Narratives are the only means by which people can communicate what goes on inside them and what links them to others. Personal narratives are "the most internally consistent interpretation of presently understood past, experienced present and anticipated future" (Cohler, 1982, p. 207).

Narrative research projects are grounded in the idea that identity is organized narratively.[2] How facts, ideas, events, or experi-

---

[2]For elaboration of the idea that identity is constructed narratively, see, among many others, Bruner (1990); Eakin (2008); MacIntyre (2007); McAdams, Josselson, and Lieblich (2001, 2006); Polkinghorne (1988); and Sarbin (1986).

ences are selected, assembled, and formulated into a story may teach us something about the narrator's sense of self and the culture in which that self is situated. Institutions and organizations are also constructed in narratives that depict how people represent the institutions they take part in, as well as their own places in the social groups of which they are a part (Linde, 2008). Narratives may be of varying length—whole life biographies or "small stories" (Bamberg, 2006) of episodes—but they represent something about how aspects of experience are linked, organized, and made personally meaningful. In narrative research, we assume that whatever stories are told have emotional and psychological truth. We have no way of assessing whether events recounted are in some way factually true (in the sense that they could be corroborated by someone else), but this is not fundamentally our concern. Whatever is experienced has some truth.

The purpose of the interview in qualitative inquiry is to create a conversation that invites the telling of narrative accounts (i.e., stories) that will inform the research question. In order to elicit the stories that will constitute the data for the project, one has to create a situation, an interview, in which someone is willing to tell personal life stories to a stranger. This is a rather unusual event, if you step back and think about it. Why would someone disclose meaningful, intimate stories to a stranger? People have a variety of motivations for agreeing to participate in such an unusual situation—a wish to be helpful to a researcher, curiosity about what such an experience might be like, or a wish to tell their stories, especially if they feel aggrieved or pained in some way. These are the conscious motives that may impel a person to consent to an interview. Less conscious, perhaps out of awareness, is the deep need to be understood that marks every human encounter. And this wish, however faint it may be, also powers the interview situation: If only someone could/ would fully understand.

What interviewees tell depends on what, or actually whom, they find when they get to the interview itself. If they find an interviewer who assures their safety from exposure and who is accepting and manages to understand well enough, most participants in (good) interviews find themselves surprised that they told what they did—usually much more than they thought they would on their way to the interview. A good interview results from the emotional and psychological interaction between researcher and participant. When people are reasonably assured that what they disclose is confidential, and they then feel the interest and acceptance of the interviewer, they usually warm to the situation and take the opportunity to speak at a depth that may be quite surprising to them. Sometimes this is called the "stranger on the train" phenomenon, in which one can speak one's heart to someone not a part of one's life—someone to whom one can disclose without consequences. But the stranger has to be able to listen.

The active engagement of listening invites the participant to discuss the depth and complexity of his or her experience. From this point of view, the aim of the interview is to obtain contextualized accounts of participants' experience, rather than "information." (I growl fiercely at students who talk about getting "information" from their interviewees. The researcher may ask, outside the boundaries of the narrative interview, for demographic details, but the material of the actual interview is *not* in any sense information.) In a good interview, the interviewee is seeking recognition from the researcher, wishing to be known as a full human being rather than as a repository of facts.

Life experience is stored in memory in the form of stories, and, asked to describe their experiences in an open-ended way, people will respond with narratives. These stories, and the meanings each participant has made of them, are what will constitute the "data" to be analyzed for the research report. These are, of course, only a sampling or subset of all the stories the participant might have told. Which stories are brought forth (and how they are told) in an interview will depend on the context of the telling. The relationship co-created in the interview situation defines that context and is influenced by how the interviewer is perceived by the interviewee, how the interview is framed, and what the interview's objectives as interpreted by the interviewee are (see also Mishler, 1986).

The realities of life are socially constructed through culture mediated by language. One of the great benefits of qualitative research is that a researcher has the opportunity to be in direct contact with a participant's language; the nature of the discourse and the communication provides a crucial opening into the participant's experiential and social world. It is therefore centrally important to qualitative research that the interview represents the linguistic expression of the participant. *How* people speak, which words they choose, how they link ideas—all these aspects of discourse are repositories of meaning and important elements to interpret.

The Whole and the Part—and the Whole

One of the most powerful images in qualitative inquiry is that of the "hermeneutic circle." This principle of hermeneutics, or meaning making, details the idea that the whole must be understood in relation to the parts, which derive their meanings from our understanding of the whole—an interpretation that then furthers our grasp of the meanings of the parts, and so on. The interpretive process is thus circular.[3] A holistic account, the aim of narrative research, must attend to the intricate relationship of the whole and the parts, recognizing that they are mutually constitutive. When we enter the interview situation, we know about neither the whole nor the parts, but our understanding of both will be building simultaneously—and our understanding will grow when we take the text back to our workspaces and analyze it.

The process of building a whole from the parts (and making sense of the parts in relation to the whole) begins when we first encounter a participant. Who is this person, and how can we learn

---

[3]Gadamer (1975) and Lyotard (1984) set out the essentials of postmodernism, which is the epistemological grounding for research from a hermeneutic stance. See also Josselson (2004) and Messer et al. (1988).

from his or her experiences? And who are we who are doing the learning? In all sciences, we recognize that to observe something is to change it. Therefore, we ask ourselves how the interviewing situation itself affects what our participants tell us. We are a part of the hermeneutic circle. The interview situation is the context of the production of the narrative and must be itself a site of interpretation and reflection.

As we understand our participants better as the interview progresses, we also recognize more clearly the reasons for their responding to the interview in the ways that they do, which in turn influence what they tell us. And our responses to them also shape what they are willing or able to reveal—a process we understand better as we learn more about how they may be experiencing us in the interaction. Indeed, there are many circularities in this process (and in this book). The interview itself has to be understood in context—both the social context and the moment-to-moment details of what is taking place between interviewer and participant. The art of interviewing does not lend itself to "first this, then that"; the parts influence the whole, which influences the parts.

The narrative interview has been conceived as a collaboration or partnership, one that empowers and does not objectify the participant (Fine, 1994). There have been lengthy scholarly discussions about the ways in which true collaboration is or is not possible, but the fundamental idea here is to follow rather than to lead participants in their detailing of their experiences (Atkinson et al., 2001; Denzin & Lincoln, 2011). The interview has also been cast as a performance or a conversation (Kvale, 1996). Kvale offers the collaborative metaphor of the researcher as a *traveler*—a person who journeys through another place and brings back to a scholarly audience tales of what he or she has learned about the lives of people there.

I would offer another metaphor, which is the interview as *dance*.[4] In this image, the researcher tries to follow the motion of the inter-

---

[4]Janesick (2010) uses the dance metaphor as a way of doing oral history interviews.

viewee, mirroring the steps the interviewee/dancer performs. Much of the massive literature on interviewing debates the context and form of asking questions. My approach to interviewing describes a way of *moving with* the participant and trying to ask as few questions as possible.

Co-Construction of the Interview

Most writers who have thought carefully about the interview as a means of doing qualitative research develop the idea that the interview is "co-constructed." What does this mean? The reflection that all interviews are co-constructed implies that the material produced by the interviewee is influenced by the context of the interview and the responses of the interviewer, so that one cannot reify the interview material as "the" story; it is only "a" story produced for the occasion of the interview. (This does not imply that it is not meaningful.) Furthermore, the interpreted meanings that are later gleaned from the material gathered in the interview are in part derived from what the interviewee says the meanings are and in part from what the interviewer/researcher understands them to suggest. These interpretations are not co-constructed (usually) in the interview in the sense of verbally negotiated understandings. Instead, they are derived inductively (by the researcher) from narratives produced in the interview, with a recognition that the narrative material itself could only have been produced in that particular interview under those particular circumstances. An interview is the coming together of two subjectivities, and an adequate analysis of and report of an interview must recognize that the content to which the interview refers is shaped by the intersubjective context.

The paradox here is that once the interview gets underway, the content of what is discussed refers to experiences outside the interview itself—events, memories, or attitudes that occurred at another time or place. This focuses the researcher's attention outside the interview situation, and it becomes easy to forget that the interviewer's responses are shaping what can be told and how it will be told (Briggs, 1986). The complexity of conducting an interview results from the necessity of the interviewer's paying attention to *both* the content and process of the interview at the same time. Although the interviewer will have time when analyzing the interview to reflect further on his or her role in producing the interview material in the way it was presented, the interviewer must have some awareness of the developing intersubjective research relationship as it is unfolding, if only to try to make necessary corrections in order to maximize the richness and depth of material that will be offered.

In the process of the interview, the interviewer has maximal impact in terms of opening areas of experience for discussion and shutting them down. This is where the co-construction in the actual dance of the interview is most notable. So often, in reviewing a transcript, a student may tell me that "Mr. Smith didn't want to talk about this aspect of his life." When we look closely at the transcript, however, we can see that the interviewer (usually unconsciously) actually closed off the discussion of that aspect of the story. If there is a main theme to this book, it is meant to offer ways of staying open to all possible aspects of the dance, and of hearing both the music and the words.

Situating the Interview Conceptually

An interview that serves narrative (qualitative) research is an open-ended invitation to someone to talk to us about some topic that interests us as researchers, and thereby to create data for us so that we may learn more about some aspect of the psychological or social world that our participant inhabits and represents. We set the boundaries of such a conversation by declaring our purpose and orienting the talk to a particular realm of experience, and then we use our skills to try to encourage the production of an authentic and personal account.

Human experience is layered and complex. Behind every story told about an experience is another story, with different shadings of and linkages to the first. Narrative conventions lead people to tell just one story at a time, but if we investigate further, we find that their stories are layered and intertwined with other stories of their lives. Narrative research is aimed at exploring such complexity. It attempts to shine a light on the linkages of the stories that construct a life and an identity—the weaving of threads that make up life experiences.

People can, of course, simplify their experience to respond to multiple-choice or short-answer questions about their lives. If I ask you to respond "True" or "False" to a questionnaire item that says, "I would like the life of a prophet,"[5] you would probably comply, but I would have no idea what is in your mind: How do you think of life as a prophet, and what about this life do you imagine would or would not seem appealing to you? (And did you think I was asking playfully or seriously? So was your response playful or serious?) I can tabulate the results across people, but I would learn nothing about the meanings you make, because I have no way to ask you. Narrative research, though, gives me an opportunity to ask. It aims to be holistic rather than reductionistic. It tries to analyze the complexity rather than to diminish it. In order for such analysis to take place, a researcher must first obtain, through an interview, a narration of experience as it is internally represented. The researcher aims to have as analyzable data stories from a life that will make possible interpretation at a variety of levels.[6] The goal is to create an interview situation in which people feel free to articulate their experience in all of its multiplicity—the feelings and thoughts that accompany important moments in their lives or aspects of themselves. A good narrative research interview makes a frame for intimate sharing, for exploration of the inner world that is situated in the participant's social reality. Narrative researchers are interested in the coming together of the individual life and the particularities of

---

[5]This is taken from a marvelous book of satire edited by Glenn Ellenbogen (1987).

[6]Some psychodynamically oriented qualitative researchers are interested in analyzing unconscious processes revealed in research interviews (Hollway & Jefferson, 2000; Clarke &Hoggett, 2009).

the social world as it is experienced, with its expectations and limitations. Each individual has a stock of unique memories and encounters that have significance for him or her, from the person's earliest moments in the family to later efforts to actualize a self within the social fabric.

If we want to understand our participants' experiences in their own terms, we have to invite their narratives and get out of the way as much as possible, except to encourage elaboration and extension. At the same time, we must recognize that participants are creating narratives *for us* and shaping them according to their assessments of who we are and how we are responding to them. The research relationship, then, becomes the context of the narrative account, and whatever we do to create the circumstances and exert control in the interview shapes what is tellable and how it will be told. If, as interviewers, we think of ourselves as askers of questions, our participants will give us answers framed in terms of our questions. If, however, we think of ourselves as (highly particular) catalysts for and recipients of stories, we will elicit the narration of stories and the meanings of these stories to our participants.

In the rest of this book, I consider how to create and maintain a research relationship with an interviewee that will maximize the possibilities of the sharing of personally meaningful stories in relation to the research question.

CHAPTER 2

Introduction to the Research Relationship

Qualitative interviewing demands personal engagement rather than formulaic responses. As researchers and interviewers, we inevitably bring ourselves to each interview encounter, and this is to be valued rather than disavowed. The fully human encounter with participants is what enables people to tell us the often intimate details of their biographies and psychological states. The idea of the neutral interviewer is a myth. Robots could not produce the kind of material for analysis that human interviewers elicit. Therefore, rather than pretending that we can sweep away the dynamics of interaction and blind ourselves to our full participation in the interview process, it is important that we instead attend to the relational and emotional interchange that takes place as we "collect" qualitative data.

When you step across the threshold into the interview itself, you will have the thrill (and terror) of encountering the unknown. You cannot know what will happen or what you may experience, let alone what you might learn. If you are sincere about learning and can open yourself to not-knowing, you can regard what will take place as an unfamiliar territory to explore, and you will take home rich data to puzzle through and analyze later. If you are too anxious about the unknown, you will try to structure the interview so that the participant's experience falls into the familiar categories you brought through the door with you. You will still take home data, but you will restrict the possibility of learning something new. Crossing the threshold into the interview also involves opening yourself to emotional experiences that you cannot predict but will have to manage, and to a relationship with the interviewee that will both shape the interaction and continue in both of your minds after you have said goodbye.

Inception of the Relationship

An interview is a meeting between two people for the purpose of one person sharing personal experience with the other. In narrative interviewing, the research relationship is central to what will be disclosed and must be attended to at each point in the research process.

From the very beginning of your project, before you even decide who you want to interview, you must steep yourself in an *ethical attitude* (Josselson, 2007) toward your participants. This means not just knowing "the rules," but making ethics a part of you.

Beyond any consideration of our research goals, we must treat our participants with respect, sensitivity, and tact. Our hope as researchers is that the experience of being interviewed in our research project will be a good experience for our participants—and certainly not a harmful one. In general, people who have taken part in a person-centered interview find it a meaningful and positive experience. For one thing, there is a sense of validation in being well listened to for an extended period of time. Being heard and accepted is all too rare in human life. Some scholars have argued that greater personal integration ensues from telling one's story in an extended, reflective way (Miller, 1996; Rosenwald, 1996), and this seems borne out by my own experience. Indeed, in my longitudinal study of women's identity, which involved interviewing women at 12-year intervals over 35 years, busy women willingly made blocks of 4 hours available (and sometimes traveled long distances) to meet with me to be interviewed again. Most valued the experience enough to go to some trouble to repeat it.

People usually find that reflecting on themselves with an attentive listener who is trying to understand their experience is inherently valuable. Many use the opportunity to explore and put into words aspects of themselves that have perhaps been in the shadows. They reflect on themselves and make new meanings, often even after the interview, as they review privately what they have said. Talking in the context of a relationship allows for a sense of the significance of their experience. They have a witness; they are known. As a researcher, you need do no more than express gratitude for the participants' openness and willingness to share their lives with you.

It is mandatory to be able to guarantee your participants anonymity (i.e., you will never use their names or the names of people in their lives) and confidentiality (i.e., you will not disclose anything about them that could be traced to them). You must also make clear that your participants are free to withdraw from your study at any time, including during the interview.

You must approach your participants with respect and integrity, and must do everything you can to preserve their dignity. I return to issues of ethics in Chapter 6.

The Relationship in the Mind

Next, you must take stock of yourself in terms of what you are bringing to the relationship that is about to begin. What drew you to this question? What are your assumptions and preconceptions about the phenomena you want to study and the people who embody these phenomena? What in your own life experience are you bringing to the study? How do you expect to feel about the people you will talk to? How do you expect them to feel toward you? Reflecting on these questions will give you some idea about what you are importing into the project and to the people you will meet. Write down your thoughts about these questions at the beginning of a private journal that you will keep throughout the project to record your evolving thoughts, feelings, and experiences.[1]

The research *relationship* begins for the researcher as soon as the researcher imagines the kinds of people he or she would like to interview as "experts" on whatever topic is the focus of the research. Usually the researcher imagines someone who represents the issues of interest to the research—a survivor of a tornado, a teacher in an inner-city school, a person who has escaped from domestic violence, a chief executive officer (CEO) in a family business, a multiracial teenager, someone living with cancer—anyone whose life story may fit the questions of the research. Often the researcher has had some personal experience with the topic, and many times the researcher imagines that the participants' stories will be just like his or her own. (They won't be.) Or the researcher knows one or more people who fall into the population under study (perhaps family members, friends, or colleagues at work). So there is usually already a picture in the researcher's mind—a picture that will be enlarged and corrected in the course of the research.

Recruitment

In order to carry out a study, you will have to contact likely participants—people who, by virtue of having a particular experience or fitting into a certain category, can speak about this experience, and from whom you can learn. Usually recruitment is done through personal networking; it is increasingly done through the Internet; and sometimes it is accomplished by advertising for volunteers or posting signs in places where people who fit the category will see them. If you are recruiting participants through networking, then usually you will introduce yourself to a participant by mention-

---

[1]See Anderson (2011) and Janesick (2011) for more detail about how to keep such a journal.

ing the link: "Jane suggested I call you because she thought you might be willing to be interviewed for my study." If the participant agrees, then he or she enters the relationship with you through the felt contact with Jane. The participant will in some (largely unconscious) way associate Jane's characteristics with you: If Jane is kind and accepting, the participant will expect you to be as well, and will thus begin the relationship with you in a positive frame of mind. If, however, the participant has had some difficult experience with Jane (e.g., Jane recently fired him or her from a job), then the participant will approach you with caution, perhaps even suspicion. In order to begin to create a good working research relationship, it then becomes important to clarify your relationship with Jane— especially the confidentiality boundary—even at the time of the first contact on the telephone. (Although it is increasingly common to schedule interview times by email or text, I think that some voice interaction before the first meeting is a good idea, so that you and the interviewee will have some sense of what it is like to talk to one another before the interview takes place.) The point here is that the research relationship begins from the first point of interaction and frames the relationship that evolves.

Sometimes researchers interview people they have known distantly in another context—for example, a friend of a friend, a relative of a friend, someone they have met at gatherings, or a former classmate or teacher. If you have some such prior relationship with a participant, the important relational challenge will be to alter this frame and to establish yourself in the role you are now taking up: that of a researcher studying a topic in which the participant has life experience expertise. In terms of forming the research relationship, this means acknowledging the other connection in a friendly way, but moving on as smoothly as possible to the business at hand. One influence of prior association on the actual interview is that participants might be tempted to prevail on what they assume you already know. For example, they may say, "Well, you know what that community was like . . . " (You don't know *their* experience of it, though.) It is important to look out for these assumptions so that you don't overlook the distinctiveness of the participants' experience. In other words, while it may be helpful to use familiarity and personal connection to enlist participants, you will need to be especially careful not to let this familiarity get in the way during the interview process.

Sometimes my students come to me wanting to interview people they know—usually relatives or their own students. I understand why they are making these requests: These are people who are near at hand, and people about whom they already know something that they think will be interesting to report or analyze. Although I know that some published studies have included or focused on the researchers' family members or students, I don't allow my own students to do this. I think that the existence of this type of prior relationship so strongly colors what can be told that the contextual analysis of the interview is saturated with this dynamic. Preserving the outside real relationship will always be more salient than the interview relationship, for both researcher and participant. One student of mine taught yoga when she wasn't studying psychology, and she wanted to interview her students about the meaning of yoga in their lives. Why would this be problematic? First of all, her yoga students would probably be wanting to tell a story emphasizing that what she taught was meaningful, and gratifying her need to feel like a good teacher. Second, she would be exposing herself to the risk of hearing intimate details of her students' lives, which she would then have to manage after the interview when she was back in the more formal teacher–student relationship. This kind of dilemma would best be handled by my student's finding another yoga teacher whose students might be willing to participate in her study, and then inviting them to volunteer. Especially if there is a power differential, an interviewer also has to be concerned about subtle coercion. On ethical grounds, this is another reason why teachers' interviewing their own students or managers' interviewing their own employees is problematic enough to make it unwise.

Volunteers

If you have recruited your participants through the Internet or through ads or posted signs, stating your research goals and what category of people you are seeking, a potential interviewee may respond by contacting you (if you have made the invitation sound friendly and inviting). You are then likely to have an extended conversation before the interview, as you verify that the volunteer indeed fits your category, and as the potential participant checks out whether you are legitimate and what your purposes are. If the person who contacts you doesn't fit the category of people you need for your study, try to be gracious as you explain the criteria that exclude him or her. In rare instances, there is some danger of unearthing troubled people in search of something you can't provide, so it is important to be cautiously alert.

Even if you offer some small payment or gift card for participation, people will volunteer for a variety of reasons, the primary one being that they want to tell their stories. This is just what you are seeking. At the same time, it is important to keep a question in your mind about what motivates each person to want to tell his or her story. This is particularly important in contextualizing the material that you will later analyze—and it may be important in the development of the research relationship. Narrative accounts are created for the circumstances in which they are told, and in this case, you are the circumstance. What do volunteers hope to achieve by volunteering? This is not a question they are likely to be able to answer directly. Most people, if asked, will say something like "It sounded like an interesting thing to do," but sometimes people will speak at the end of the interview about political motives in the sense of having some injustice or oppression heard by others. After the interview, especially as you analyze the material, the issue of volunteering at all becomes one more part of the context to be subjected to reflection.

People in institutions like shelters, retirement homes, prisons, or hospitals are most likely to respond to requests to volunteer partly to fill empty time.[2] People in support groups are also likely to respond well to requests to volunteer (or even to volunteer on their own),

---

[2]Institutional review boards (IRBs), however, often make it quite difficult to conduct research in such institutions.

because they are already seeking a better understanding of whatever life circumstance led them to the support group. Sometimes people volunteer when they are in distress and imagine that the interview may help them, like seeing a therapist.[3] They are not likely to be forthcoming about this, but in such cases you will feel the press of this dynamic during the interview.

Networked Recruitment

Studies often call for particular sorts of people who are best reached through networking—identifying suitable participants through one means or another and then inviting them (sometimes with no personal linking contact). In such cases, you will usually have to offer some persuasion to participate, especially if a participant is a busy person. You will need to communicate that there is a serious and important reason for this person to give time to the project; you will also need to distinguish yourself from a telemarketer or survey researcher. The nature of the linking contact can sometimes help, but what becomes most important is to persuade the person that he or she *in particular* is of special value to your study and that the study itself will be of special value to knowledge. One student, for example, wanted to study processes of identification in daughters of famous women, and she did a lot of preparation by thinking through how she was going to present this project to these women ("There are not that many of you; it is important to the psychology of women to know how successful women influence their daughters' identity; it would be helpful in learning about your experience

---

[3] I am not in any way suggesting that a research interview is like seeing a therapist—only that some interviewees may think that it is. At the same time, many interviewees do feel that the opportunity to tell their stories has some healing and integrating (i.e., therapeutic) aspects (Miller, 1996). James Pennebaker has also demonstrated empirically over many studies that the telling of narratives can reduce the effects of trauma (Pennebaker & Seagal, 1999; Pennebaker & Chung, 2007).

for people who counsel others in the same situation; it will be completely anonymous and confidential, and you will have an opportunity to make sure that your mother's identity cannot be guessed," etc.). In such circumstances, it is important to emphasize the fundamental structure of the research relationship (the participants are the experts, you are the learner; they will be making a contribution to knowledge), and also to emphasize that you have a particular interest in these *particular* participants because of some special characteristic you know about them already. In other words, your request has to be personal and humble to enlist participation. After a good experience, such a participant may know—and then be willing to suggest—others who might also be suitable for the research. (This is known as "snowballing.")

In some cases, networked recruitment can pose particular ethical challenges, such as when several people from the same community take part in a study. This can complicate issues of anonymity and disguise.[4]

The Challenge of Meeting, and the Dilemmas of Seeing and Being Seen

Before I discuss actually meeting your participant, I want to back up and consider the general relational dynamics of meeting. When two people meet, they form instantaneous impressions of one another. Both people know that this is taking place, but they usually refrain from calling attention to it. In order to understand the relational dynamics of the interview situation, we have to consider what it means for people to be looking at and thinking about each other. Both being observed and observing others carry distinct but often intense anxieties. To increase my workshop participants' sensitivities to these issues, I ask them to engage in a 1-minute exercise in which two people stand facing one another and are asked just to

[4]See Lieblich (1996) for a full discussion of these issues.

look at the other person without speaking. (I encourage you to find a partner and try it. See Exercise 1 below.) This exercise usually and lays bare the deep and pervasive anxieties that attend looking and being looked at—which, after all, constitute the essence of what takes place in an interview. As a matter of social custom, of course, people don't usually do this in social situations. In fact, people are socialized to speak (often in relatively meaningless "small talk") to cover the anxieties of what is actually taking place: looking at and being looked at; being taken in by each other and simultaneously forming a (hidden) mental idea of each other. Understanding these anxieties, though, helps a researcher recognize the delicate negotiations that are taking place interpersonally in the interview dance.

Exercise 1. A Minute of Looking

Find a partner and a device to time 1 minute. Stand facing one another. The task will be, when the time begins, to observe one another without speaking or making sounds. When the minute is over, each of you (without speaking) takes a notepad and writes down all the feelings you were aware of during the exercise, as well as what you observed of your partner. It is important to write down these feelings and observations, because they are instantaneous and fleeting.

In the workshop, after people have had time to observe one another and to write their experiences, the whole group reassembles to discuss, in turn, how it felt to be observed and how it felt to observe. After this discussion, the partners in each pair should take 10 minutes to talk to one another about what each person observed, and to try to understand any observations that one or the other may have felt did not fit their experience. This can be a way of ferreting out projections and provide useful feedback to the participants in the exercise about their spontaneous and unexamined ways of thinking about others.

In the review of this exercise, I ask my students to try to articulate what was anxiety-provoking about being looked at. Many say that they felt uncomfortable, embarrassed, and self-conscious. Some can articulate a sense of vulnerability, like being naked. At the same time, some people speak about feeling excited by and enjoying the attention. Some are aware of wanting to impress the person who was looking at them, and most can recognize a concern with what the observer was thinking. Most are aware of wondering what they were presenting to be seen by the other person.

These dynamics are present in every interview situation. Self-consciousness is consciousness of self, and focus on the self of the participant is the aim of every interview. The participant, the one under observation, is aware of the researcher's gaze and wonders (and tries to divine) what the researcher may be thinking about him or her. The one being observed is often vigilant about the direction of the observer's gaze: What is the observer looking at? What captures his or her attention? As my students and I pursue the analysis of the exercise further, we discover that the underlying fear is of shame—of being found wanting, of the other's seeing aspects of the self that are hated and usually well hidden. The shame derives from the fear that something "bad" in the self is being seen. For some, the fear is more like fear of being judged, which is related to but not identical with shame.

All of these reactions share a concern with what might be going on in the observer. What evokes anxiety is not knowing what the other person might be thinking. The experience of being looked at, at least in Western culture, is socially connected to shame. Think about what happens in a theatre if someone is talking during the performance. Others turn and look at the person; the act of looking itself indicates that the behavior is inappropriate. Similarly, many people were raised by parents who signaled their disapproval by looking at them intently. Staring at someone is how we socially shame others. So being seen is, at many levels, perilously close to the possibility of shame. The experience of being observed carries with it these anxieties: "What are they really thinking about what they see of me, and are they seeing my shameful parts?"

Paradoxically, at the same time, people harbor a deep wish to be seen, and this too can feel like a shameful wish. (Thus, those who were aware of enjoying the attention in the exercise often felt embarrassed disclosing this.) The wish, though, is to be seen as we see ourselves. We long to be known by others, known as we know ourselves. We wish to see ourselves in the mirror of others' eyes.

All of these reactions are taking place at some level in the interview situation. The interviewer must be aware of the risks of shame that are involved, and correspondingly must master an accepting, respectful attitude. Acceptance of the other person as he or she is constitutes the antidote to shame. When interviewers speak of "making the other person comfortable," they are usually referring to interpersonal moves aimed at reducing the possibility of shame. Sensitive interviewers are aware of themselves as people who *look* (much as in this exercise), and they titrate their gaze to the comfort of each participant, finding the right amount of looking—not too penetrating, not too superficial. They must look at the participant in a way that conveys interest and recognition, but not intrusion—and never anything that might be shaming. They must remain aware that the participant is continually having an internal conversation about what it might be safe to reveal.

Since this exercise is designed to unveil the anxieties of observation and hold onto them long enough to experience them, we can also witness the psychological defenses people employ to suppress these anxieties. Some people in my workshops notice that they made themselves feel invisible; they told themselves that the observer couldn't really see them or see anything important about them. Some describe keeping their focus on observing as a way to quell the anxieties about being seen. The interview analogue to these processes is the effort not to reveal anything too personal, to talk but remain essentially hidden, to try to direct the observer/interviewer's gaze to less tender areas of the self. Many interviews begin with this defensive stance but become more genuine when, as the feelings of acceptance in the relationship build, the dangers of feeling shame may feel less threatening.

The Dynamics of Observing

The act of observing is accompanied by its own particular anxieties. When we attend to the anxieties of observing in this exercise, people become even more animated. Workshop participants describe being afraid of harming the other with their gaze. The act of looking at another arouses repressed primitive voyeuristic urges and anxieties—fears of seeing what one is not allowed to see, and fears that looking itself can be aggressive. Many speak of experiencing a dilemma about where to look; they wondered whether they could look beyond what was most apparent (e.g., by looking too long at one part of their partner's body), or were fearful that they might see something different from what was intended. Participants in the exercise describe becoming anxious if they felt they were intruding, penetrating, or violating some boundary. Others note a fear that they were looking at something they were not supposed to see or going somewhere forbidden. A person in one workshop spoke of fearing to see that her partner had something stuck in her teeth! Many people describe feeling very distressed when they perceived signs of discomfort in the other and worried that they were the cause of the discomfort.

One striking aspect of this exercise is the difficulty in locating some of these feelings. Many participants described perceiving that their partners were very uncomfortable, but the same partners denied having felt any discomfort. Some people told their partners, "I was trying to make you feel comfortable," only to have their partners respond, "But I wasn't uncomfortable about being looked at. I was busy looking at you." In these replays, we are able to see how easily one person can project anxiety onto the other, and how readily observers tried to manage their own anxiety about observing by treating it as anxiety in the one observed.

In the workshop, we wonder together what it means to "make someone comfortable." How do we manage other people's feelings for them? Is this just a cover for making ourselves comfortable—and, if so, to reduce which anxieties? In the observation exercise, these dynamics seem to go like this:

I perceive anxiety here. Perhaps it is the threat of shame that you are feeling, so I will do some things to indicate that I am friendly, am not a threat, and do not intend to judge you. Doing these things also makes me feel less anxious about the part of me that may be intrusive or may indeed be judging you, but I am ashamed of this and don't want you to see it.

In other words, the anxieties are intertwined, and making the other "comfortable" is aimed at the observer's own anxieties as well. This would imply that as we become less anxious in our role as interviewers/observers in an actual study, those we interview will be (and seem to us) less anxious as well.

There are strong individual differences here (and the anxieties of looking and being looked at are more intense for opposite-sex pairs). Looking at someone and being looked at set off unconscious associations as well as culturally encoded meanings that we have to become aware of. Looking is intimate and may feel erotic to the one who is looking and/or the one who is the object of the gaze. (This is equally true of self-disclosure.) Some potential interviewers have more anxiety about looking, others about being looked at. Some people describe defending themselves against the anxieties of being looked at by pretending to themselves that they were not being observed and focusing just on observing. Others describe being afraid to see anything of their partners and mainly looking away. Talking about these experiences helps workshop participants clarify which particular anxieties are most salient for them, how they defend themselves, and therefore which dynamics they are most likely to bring to the interview situation.

This exercise serves to make interviewers more aware of the emotional temperature on both sides of looking and being looked at. This is often misread, but the misreading itself can be explored in the context of the exercise. Everyone struggles with how to look openly but with respect, and this is indeed the goal of the stance of the research relationship.

In the interview situation, an interviewer and a participant are looking at each other all the time. If they put words on top of it, they become less aware that all this is going on, but the dynamics are still operating beneath the surface. The two people in the interview situation are observing each other and forming pictures of the other. It is *not* just you, the interviewer, who is observing the interviewee. It is *also* the interviewee who is observing you, the interviewer, and noticing what you wear, how you sit, when you smile, how you respond, and how your minute facial movements indicate your feelings about what you are hearing. The interviewee is making judgments about who you are, and this may not correspond to who you think you are.

An interviewer who is very anxious about being observed will have to learn to bear the increased consciousness of self as the interviewee tries to make sense of who the interviewer is by looking and observing. If self-consciousness in the interviewer is too great, the interviewer works to protect him- or herself from the exposure and becomes more concerned with feeling secure in the interview situation than attending to the participant. If anxiety about looking is too great, the interviewer backs off from disclosures that may signal emotional arousal and moves away lest the *interviewer* have to bear discomfort.

In the intersubjective dance that is the interview situation, the interviewer must have sufficient training and supervision to monitor and manage his or her anxiety and other emotional responses enough to be able to sit with and contain the affective experience that may arise during the interview (in both the interviewee and in him- or herself). In my workshops, I invite participants to imagine what they are most afraid of happening in an interview. The most common question posed to me is this: "What should I do if an interviewee gets upset, or even cries, during an interview?" I usually point out that if the participant is not comfortable in the interview situation, he or she will not be expressing deeply felt emotions. As in the exercise, the interviewer is afraid of seeing something he or she is not supposed to see—but, after all, it is the interviewee who is overtly expressing intense feelings. People do not tell anyone anything they do not want to tell; an interviewer cannot *make* anyone share personal feelings or experiences. The issue is being able to bear it. When people talk of emotionally powerful experiences, which are often the topics of narrative research, they may feel intensely or talk about things that are hard for you, the interviewer, to hear. You have to be ready for this and not run away in fear.

The second most common anxiety is that there will be silence, and the interviewer will "not know what to say." I address this worry later in this book, but the short response is that if an interviewer is moving in sync with an interviewee, silence will not be a problem. The third highest-ranking anxiety is "What if my inexperience shows?" This is a reflection of the anxieties about shame that I have alluded to earlier. Indeed, there is exposure to shame in the interview situation, and as an interviewer you will have to find ways to manage it. A bit of fumbling or uncertainty is not really a terrible thing, as long as you stay focused on your interest in the interviewee. If the interviewee can see or sense your anxiety, it is not a problem; it will just make the interviewee less anxious in turn.

Preparing Yourself for the Interview

Who You Are

Reflexivity involves an attempt to recognize your own assumptions or preconceived ideas about the person or narratives that you are about to encounter. The effort is to create an open, receptive mind that can receive the impact of the participant's experience, and this involves clearing out whatever preexisting thoughts or attitudes may be cluttering the listening path. This is, of course, an ideal. As soon as you have to respond to the participant, you will be bringing aspects of yourself to the interaction. The reflexive attitude becomes one of noticing what you *are* doing in the interaction, rather than trying to maintain the illusion that you are doing nothing at all. Your various responses to your interviewee—the words you choose, your tone of voice, whether you smile—will tell both you and the participant something about who you are. Reflecting on your own reactions is how you can learn about your presumptions. If, for example, you feel shocked by something you hear from your interviewee, you can learn something about what you consider social taboos or what narratives you have implicitly expected to hear (Sands & Krumer-Nevo, 2006), even if you do a good job of not showing that you were taken aback.

In order to practice a reflexive stance as a researcher, you must find a quiet time and place, and try to assess meditatively whatever thoughts or preconceptions appear in your mind. How does your own social location in terms of gender, race, class, age, sexual orientation, or nationality inform how you think about your research question? What previous understandings have you come to from the literature you have read? What expectations do you have of what you might hear? How do you locate the person you are about to encounter in the context of the people you have already known in your life? What aspects of your own life draw you to this study? What is your emotional investment in it? What are your fantasies about what you might discover and the impact this might have on the world? What anxieties do you have about working with this particular group of participants? How do you expect them to respond to you?

Writing in a journal is very useful in this process and serves to document the evolution of your thinking about the research topic. Rosemary Anderson's (2011) intuitive approach to qualitative research makes this a mandated part of the research process; she advocates using dreams and associations to try to locate your intuitive preconceptions of the topic at hand. Your task as an interviewer is to try to keep as open a mind as possible, to allow new impressions and ideas to enter. Opening the mind means in part achieving clarity about what is already there.

Besides reflecting on the personal assumptions and biases you are bringing to the interview, it is important to reflect on your orientation to the whole process. The ideal structure of the interview is a keen awareness that the participant is the expert here, rather than you. The participant is the expert on his or her own experience. The necessary stance is that you as the researcher are ignorant: "I know nothing about your experience; that's why I want you to tell it to me." Giving over the "expert" role is sometimes difficult for interviewers (particularly neophyte researchers) who want to be recognized for their knowledge and expertise.

The aim of the interview is to understand the participant's experience as fully as possible without judgment or interference. This is sometimes a hard shift for clinical psychologists, counselors, people in medical helping professions, or sometimes teachers, who are accustomed to hearing people's experiences but to listening with some idea of changing the persons or fixing their "problems." In a research interview, such intervention is completely inappropriate, and people who work in helping roles must learn to listen in a different way—to hear without thinking about how to change things.

For those who come to this work without a history of helping roles, the initial dynamics are different. These researchers are often worried about getting too intimate, hearing strong emotional expressions, or getting "too personal." They don't have reflex reactions to "help," but they have to find ways to bring themselves to hear whatever a participant wishes to tell.

As the interviewer, you have to prepare to enter each research relationship tolerating uncertainty and being ready to reflect on your own feelings and experiences as these emerge in the interview. Whatever occurs in the interview will be something to learn from. Enter each relationship with hope, receptivity, and focused curiosity. Inevitably, some interviews go better than others, but learning is possible no matter what. Expectations of yourself that are too high can also be crippling.

Who the Participant Thinks You Are

As the research relationship begins, it is important for you as the researcher to recognize that while you have some preconceived idea of who the participant "is," the participant also has some picture of who you "are." This will be manifested at many levels of the interview conversation that will take place and will change over its course. At the beginning, it is most important to be reasonably certain that the interviewee understands what you are doing there. People have different ideas about research and what you might do with the material, and all this should be discussed at the outset. Having participants sign a consent form is not a substitute for this conversation.

Depending on whom you are interviewing, the participant group may or may not understand what "research" is. When I was interviewing Ethiopians who had immigrated to Israel, I had to do a lot of discussing to explain that I was not a journalist. There were some participants (nonstudents) who understood about journalism but not about university researchers, even though we were meeting in my university office. (In fact, it wasn't so easy to explain the difference.) Some of my participants had felt wounded in the past by journalists (or knew people who had), and I had to provide a simple explanation of my research into how people valued their relationships with one another and the ways in which it would help people who thought about and taught psychology to better understand people from different cultures. I had to explain that I intended to write about what I learned, but not in newspapers or magazines—rather, in special books that people who worked in universities might read. Usually participants' questions in regard to the research enterprise have to do with what you are going to do with their stories. You have to explain this fully, especially with regard to anonymity, confidentiality, and whatever role you will be giving them in deciding about what might be made public.

Other people may come as participants expecting that they will be in some kind of laboratory experiment, or that there is some hidden purpose or deception involved. If you are interviewing people within an organization, you will often have to overcome the worry that you are a spy for management. Sometimes, if it is a community you are studying, people are concerned about how you might portray their community. Often this occurs if a community feels it has been badly portrayed or misrepresented by some prior researchers. You cannot, of course, promise at the outset what you will report. In such circumstances, though, you can express your hope to produce a fuller and more understanding portrait of the community—or you can find a way to involve the community in decisions about what to publish and how, even if part of the publication involves a response to or critique of your findings.

Sometimes an interview is well underway before you understand better whom a participant thinks he or she is talking to. Molly Andrews (2007) reports that while interviewing people about their political activism, she realized with great surprise toward the end of one interview that the audience her East German participant was addressing was "uncomprehending people in the West," a position that Molly did not feel matched her own perception of herself. Narrations are always addressed to an audience, and the audience in the mind of the participant may not be the "you" that you are to yourself. Or they may think they are talking to others through you. We researchers often do not know at the outset what categories of "us" and "them" are salient for our participants—or whether they regard us as part of "us" or as some "them" that we hadn't expected to count ourselves among. During (or after) interviews, reflecting on who we are to our participants can lead to a richer understanding of the contexts in which they construct their lives.

All participants enter the research relationship wondering who you are and why you are interested in them. Their larger interest may be in what you may do with the stories they tell you, but not all interviewees are very interested in this. All interviewees are, however, concerned about whether or not you are enough like them to be able to understand them, for this will shape what it will feel like to talk to you. If you and a participant are very different in group membership, then you will have to rely on your shared humanity as a basis for understanding.

Sometimes interviewees are suspicious that you are making money from their stories, and you may need to address this. Many researchers have commented on the ways in which we academics do indeed make use of people's life stories for our own career advancement. If this issue is raised in the relationship, your response must, of course, be straightforward.

The question often arises about whether or not to tell participants that you are (or are not) a member of the group you are studying. This is a complex question. Perhaps most important is to make a carefully considered decision about whether or not to declare your membership in the group and to examine your motives for doing so. On the one hand, it seems that declaring that you are gay, a survivor of domestic abuse, even "also a teacher," or the like would form a bond and ease participants' fears of being judged or not understood. On the other hand, no two people's experiences are alike, and declaring that you are "the same" may seem as if it subtracts from the uniqueness of the participants' experiences—as though they can only disclose what they imagine they have in common with you. Or they feel they have to narrate their own experience in light of what they imagine to be your experience. In addition, groups have subgroups, and sometimes sharing a larger group membership evokes within-group prejudices (e.g., "Well, maybe you were once in a cult, but nothing like *my* cult"). My advice in such situations is not to lead off with self-disclosure about being a member of the group. Some participants may ask you directly at some point in the interview about your group membership, and if this happens, I think you need to answer honestly and simply, in as general a way as possible without seeming evasive.

This general rule of thumb, like most general rules about managing the interviewing process, can get complicated and has exceptions. I was supervising a doctoral student who was studying the experience of women who had been raped, but she did not want it widely known that she herself had been raped. If she were to disclose this to her participants, then she would have to report it in her dissertation, which would be published, and all the world would then know about it. She would then be sacrificing in regard to herself the anonymity that she was guaranteeing her participants. What to do? We finally settled on her deciding to say, if asked, that she felt she was close enough to such a terrible experience to be able to understand the many feelings that being raped might engender. In this way, we felt that she was responding to the central underlying question, which was not about a question of fact. Rather, the question was about whether or not she could understand.

Entering the Research Relationship: Overview

The research relationship is fundamentally a special case of a human relationship, and we have to be thoughtful about the relationship dynamics that are being created between us and our participants. Throughout this book, as throughout the research process, we have to pay attention at all times both to the content of what is being told and to the state of the relationship in which it is being told. The two are inseparable: The relationship always invites the content, and the content affects the relationship.

The interviewee will be experiencing feelings both about the encounter with the interviewer and about the biographical stories that come to mind and are (or are not) being narrated. In terms of the relationship with the interviewer, the emotional climate of the interchange will be determined by whether the interviewee is feeling understood and accepted, or misunderstood and/or judged.

There is no way to be "neutral" or "objective" as the interviewer in such a situation. The research encounter is filled with affect—both the researcher's and the participant's. The researcher may feel, at different times in the process of interviewing, anxious, bored, sad, joyful, admiring, guilty, loving, ashamed, irritated, amused, contemptuous, or distracted. A range of feelings is to be expected and reflected on (but, if possible, not expressed). The novice interviewer will primarily be worried about whether he or she is being seen as professional and competent, or whether uncertainty or awkwardness is showing. Novice interviewers are also often uncomfortable with interviewees' sharing intimate details or expressing strong feelings. They might be tempted to respond as they might with a friend— sharing related personal stories, offering platitudinous reassurances, or expressing surprise. If they are interviewing traumatized or disadvantaged people, they may fear being overwhelmed with pity. The experienced interviewer learns to observe these reactions and to make a mental note of them for later analysis, but to maintain a stance of interested listening—trying to stay *with* the interviewee, and absorbing as much as possible how the interviewee might have thought and felt in the context of the story being related. Sometimes these experiences, when they involve intense loss or pain, are indeed hard to contain emotionally, but this is something to consider in choosing a topic. (Someone who cannot bear another's pain probably ought not to be studying people who escaped the World Trade Center on September 11, 2001, as one of my easily distressed students proposed to do. I thought she would do better with another research question.)

The research relationship that unfolds as the interview progresses creates an intersubjective field of interacting experiential worlds (Stolorow, Atwood, & Orange, 2002). What occurs as talk is not just a product of the interviewee's inner world, but a co-production of the reciprocally interacting worlds of the interviewee and the interviewer. In later chapters, I focus on how this mutual influence is manifested through the dialogue of the interview.

CHAPTER 3

Planning the Interview

The Interview's Design and Focus

The whole idea of planning the interview suggests that we must devise a structure for what we will invite our participants to talk about. But narrative interviewing is by design open-ended and unprescribed. The paradox of this approach is that the interview will be both unstructured *and* bounded. It will not be structured in the question-and-answer format that most people associate with interviews, but it will be bounded by our research question, which defines the terms of having the interview at all. The literature is replete with ideas about trying to get to know the whole person, which is in some sense true, but practically and conceptually we are trying to get to know the whole person in relation to some question that we bring to him or her. If we are studying the development of people's spiritual beliefs, for example, then their relationship to their pets would not be our focus unless *they* bring up a pet in the interview as related to their spiritual experience. Similarly, if we are studying people's relationship to their pets, spirituality may not be discussed. So, in the interest of being precise, our aim is to investigate the wholeness of the person *in relation* to some aspect of his or her experience—the aspect determined by the focus of our research.

The Questions: "Big Q," Recruitment, and "Little q"

The Big Q Question

If you are planning to do a qualitative study that relies on interviews, it is because the kind of data that you wish to obtain focuses
on some people's experience of some aspect of life, and what you
want to learn about is their experience and the meanings that they
have made of it. If you are already at the stage of planning the interview, then you have developed a conceptual question that is the
framework for your research. The conceptual question derives from
the scholarly literature and takes the next step in some scholarly
conversation. Your literature review has revealed what other scholars have to say about the question you are exploring, and your proposed research study is aimed at adding to this discussion. You have
undoubtedly spent a great deal of time articulating and specifying
your conceptual question, and this question I call the "Big Q" question. It is the question that links you to your academic colleagues,
distinguishes your study from a journalistic feature story on a related
topic, and marks the dialogue to which you will return when you
publish your finished research project.

I advise you to write your Big Q question in as large a font
as possible, print it, and paste it over your desk. Your conceptual
question is your road map. It's what you are trying to find out. You
have to have it crystal-clear in your mind. This doesn't mean that it
doesn't change over time, isn't amplified, isn't modified. But it's the
core of what you are striving to know. When you get lost in your
project (which you inevitably will), it is the anchor to which you
can return to remind you why you are doing this in the first place
and what you are trying to learn. Human experience is endlessly
complex, and most qualitative researchers have moments of feeling
overwhelmed by the layers of the complexity. The Big Q question
helps you to stay focused, to respect the diversions of the narrations
you will obtain, and to find the thread of your own interest that
forms the boundaries of your project.

Here are some examples of conceptual questions explored by my students in their dissertations:

How do men construct the work–family balance? (Simon, 2012) [Conceptual framework: Male identity.]

How do girls who have been sexually abused experience telling about their abuse? (Forrester, 2002) [Conceptual framework: Secondary trauma in disclosure.]

How do people diagnosed with bipolar disorder manage the way this disorder is socially constructed? (Goldberg, 2007) [Conceptual framework: Social construction of psychopathology.]

How do people with borderline personality disorder experience the therapeutic relationship?[1] [Conceptual framework: Relational structures in borderline personality.]

How do married women who discover lesbian attractions in adulthood rework their sexual identity?[2] How is sexuality in women "fluid"? [Conceptual framework: Sexual identity and erotic plasticity in women.]

How do young people who have lost a parent maintain a continuing bond with their dead parent? (Nasim, 2007) [Conceptual framework: The dynamics of grief.]

Note that all of these are appropriately "how" questions. They are aimed at detailing process in order to obtain a better understanding of the theoretical questions. Such questions necessitate interview-based narrative research methods. But none of these questions could be put directly as an invitation to narration. Each has to be broken down to something that is near to the participants' experience, both for recruitment and for the interview itself.

---

[1]Work in progress conducted by Shari Goldstein.

[2]Work in progress conducted by Jeanne Miller.

The Recruitment Question

You will need to enlist people to talk to you, and for this, you have to tell people what you are studying. This has to be in the form of a general statement, not technically framed in conceptual language like the Big Q question. Generally it will be phrased in terms of the specific group you are wishing to study (e.g., women who discovered in adulthood that they are lesbians, people who have been diagnosed with bipolar disorder, or people who have recovered from anorexia nervosa). In your recruitment materials, whether oral or written, you will simply say that you are doing a study of _____ people (immigrants, CEOs, chronically ill, crime victims, whatever the category may be) and trying to understand their experiences.

Use the most general category that fits, so as not to label the participants in a way that may too narrowly precategorize them or lead them to wonder why you might be singling them out. This may involve some careful thinking. One of my students wanted to study relational experience among those who were assessed to have an avoidant attachment style on a standard measure. He administered the measure to a class of college students and told the group that some would be selected for an interview. He couldn't tell people that they were classified as having an avoidant attachment style without prejudging the interview and possibly having to begin with understandable defensiveness on the part of the participants. So when he called those he selected, he simply said that he wanted to interview them about their significant relationships. No potential interviewees asked before the interview why they were selected, but he was prepared to tell those who might have asked that he was interviewing a range of people in relation to the questionnaires they had filled out. After the interview, *if people asked*, he might have explained about the attachment categories and then inquired of them in what way they thought that being classified as having an avoidant attachment style might have fit them. But this discussion could only take place after the interview.

When you are recruiting people, you need to tell them not only what sorts of people you are seeking, but what you want to know and how long it will take. So you must say that you are seeking people willing to talk to you in an interview for a specified amount of time (usually 1–3 hours) about their experiences with whatever the topic is. This statement, too, should be deliberately vague and general. There is no point in specifying details about your conceptual question, because this is not of interest to your participants. It is very important to stress that you will be interested in learning about their individual experiences with whatever you will invite them to talk about. You must also say that you will be (audio-)recording the interview in order to transcribe it later and learn from it.

Any of the conceptual questions listed above can be described to a participant as the framework for the study in simple, general language, and this is what is necessary to engage the participant. Below are examples of moving from the conceptual question to a description of the study that can be presented to participants during recruitment.

Big Q (conceptual) question	Description
How do men construct the work–family balance? [Conceptual framework: Male identity.]	I am doing a study of how men manage their work and family responsibilities, and I'd like to talk to you about how this works in your life.
How do girls who have been sexually abused experience telling about their abuse? [Conceptual framework: Secondary trauma in disclosure.]	I want to talk to the girls in this center about what it was like to first tell someone about what happened to you, about how you decided who to tell, and then about what that was like.

(*cont.*)

Big Q (conceptual) question	Description
How do people diagnosed with bipolar disorder manage the way this disorder is socially constructed? [Conceptual framework: Social construction of psychopathology.]	I want to learn about what happens to people when they are first given a diagnosis of bipolar disorder, and what then happens over time.
How do people with borderline personality disorder experience the therapeutic relationship? [Conceptual framework: Relational structures in borderline personality.]	I am studying people who have been diagnosed with borderline personality disorder and their experiences with psychotherapy.
How do married women who discover lesbian attractions in adulthood rework their sexual identity? How is sexuality in women "fluid"? [Conceptual framework: Sexual identity and erotic plasticity in women.]	I'm talking to women who discover in adulthood that they are lesbians about what this discovery was like, what they did, and how this led them to think differently about their lives and perhaps make changes.
How do young people who have lost a parent maintain a continuing bond with their dead parent? [Conceptual framework: The dynamics of grief.]	I am studying people who have lost a parent before they were 18, in order to understand the impact of this experience on their lives.

The study description question should be repeated at the time of the interview to restate what you are interested in and why you are doing this study, as well as to remind each participant of the question he or she agreed to talk to you about during the recruitment phase. Your task at this point is to talk about your study just enough so that the participant feels ready to join you in a collaborative effort to investigate it, using his or her own experience as an instance of what you are researching. The statements above are ways of telling the participant in general what you are interested in, but they are not necessarily meant to stand alone. You may need to explain or discuss them a bit, so that participants feel they understand what you are focusing on, and also that they feel that they indeed have experience from which you can learn. Your aim at this crucial moment is to bring the participant into connection with your overall question so that you are, at least to some extent, looking together in the same direction. Or, to stay with the dance metaphor, you are defining the kind of dance you will be doing. Before the interview begins, the participant should have the sense of "Oh, now I know what the interviewer is interested in." It is your task as the interviewer to monitor the participant's basic understanding of the project.

The Little q Question: Framing the Interview for the Interviewee

The "little q" question marks the launching point of the interview conversation. It is the place to begin the narration. The language of the little q question is crucially important. It must orient the interviewee and engage him or her with your research interest, but must not color the interview in a direction that doesn't fit the interviewee's experience. As the researcher, you must pay careful attention to framing the little q question so that the participant can develop the narrative along the lines of his or her own experience. It marks the place to begin.

One of the best examples of the dilemmas of the little q question came from the study of a former student, Alice Forrester, who was interested in the issue of the ways in which young girls' telling people about having been sexually abused increased or decreased the trauma. She was working in a treatment facility for sexually abused girls, so she had comfortable access to this population. Initially, she had wanted to start with this question: "Tell me about the first time you told somebody about your sexual abuse." You might pause for a moment and think about what's wrong with that question.

Beginning with asking the girl to narrate historically, starting with her first experience of telling about what had happened to her is an excellent place to start. But "sexual abuse"—whose phrase is that? It is a label that society has provided, a legal word, a categorical word. But is it the language of experience? Perhaps it is for older women, but even so, it isn't a word of lived experience; it's not a way of describing what is happening to oneself in the moment, and it is not likely that girls would use this label to "tell" about it. It is hard to imagine that any of these girls went to their parents or teachers and said, "I want to tell you about my sexual abuse." To engage the experience, Alice had to grapple with how to get into the experiential world of her participants and to engage them enough so they could bring their world to her, rather than ask them to repackage their experience in societal terms. It was necessary to find a different way to open the interview—one that would move nearer to the girls' felt experience.

What we came up with was this: "I know that something happened to you—something you thought shouldn't be happening—and that at some point you told someone about it. What do you call the thing that happened that led you to be in a facility like this?" Girls responded in a variety of ways. One said, "Well, my uncle was touching me." Another said, "My brother was doing bad things to me." One memorable girl said, "Oh, you mean the nasty?" For the rest of each interview, Alice used each girl's own words and labels to talk about the experience—and obtained very rich interviews. Once Alice had the language of each participant's experience, she could then move to the next experience-near question she planned, which was "Please tell me about the first time you told someone about it."

At the very beginning of the interview, the interviewee is wondering, "What do you want to know about *me*? What about *me* is of interest to you?" (The participant *is not* interested in your research project at this juncture.) Your opening question, then, has to give participants a bookmark in their ongoing internal life narrative, a place to pick up their story. You have to make clear which aspects of their particular experience or life story you think would be useful to hear about for your study. In other words, you have to set a starting point, one that is close to their experience.

Of course, every experience is intertwined with the larger life history context. But we can't simply ask people to tell us a whole life history. Such an idea presumes that there is some reified life story, as though somehow people have lodged in their brains a kind of file called "life story" that they can download into speech at will. In fact, a narrative interview invites a participant to create a (partial) life story on the spot, just for the research, under the circumstances that a researcher defines. This is not a loss. Generally, there are distinct neighborhoods of the life story space that the researcher wants to hear about in order to inform the research question.

Sometimes a researcher is interested in how particular experiences get woven into the life history, and to ask about them directly would disrupt the very thing the researcher wants to study. In such instances, beginning with a more general question may be preferable. For example, one researcher wanted to study memories of high school and their role in adult identity, but to ask specifically about high school experiences would shine a light in a way that would make it hard to discover the larger context. As a result, she chose for her little q question a question about most important experiences in life, and she asked her participants to tell her about the experiences they had while growing up that had the greatest influence on their becoming the kind of people they became. In this way, the researcher could then see what weight was given spontaneously to high school experiences.

The little q question has to be near to the participant's experience; it should ring bells in an area of the participant's mind that he or she is comfortable talking about at the outset. It is important to check your little q question to make sure that you are not making assumptions about the participant's experience, or directing attention immediately to "problems" you think he or she may have. One student wanted to investigate how people managed crises in family businesses and began the interview by asking about this. His interviewees seemed defensive, largely, he thought, because they were powerful people. Another possibility is that the interviewer was leading off by talking about difficulties, possibly failures. It might have been better to phrase the little q question in more neutral terms: "I'm trying to learn about what it's like to be in business with members of your family. I'd like to hear about what sorts of pleasures and challenges arise from melding these parts of your life." This kind of opening would have left the participants free to begin with either the pleasures *or* the challenges. The interviewer could always get to crises and difficulties later—and these particular participants might have needed to know that the interviewer was clearly hearing about their power and success before they could speak about the more vulnerable parts of their experience that they felt less certain about. As in learning to dance, it may be best to begin with the easier steps.

Whatever little q question you decide on, try it out on yourself. Can *you* respond to such a question? Get a colleague to interview you, beginning with this question. If you have difficulty orienting yourself to the question, you have to reframe it. (If you aren't a member of the group you are studying, modify the question somewhat. For instance, if you haven't been diagnosed with bipolar disorder, talk about something you *have* been diagnosed with—or could have been.)

Another way to approach the little q question is with some kind of drawing that delimits the life history into manageable chunks. When I wanted to study how people construct emotional meaning in their relationships over the life course, I realized that there was no simple, direct way to ask about this. I thought about asking, "Tell me about the relationships that have been most meaningful to you in your life," but when I tried it out on myself, I got immediately flooded by so many images of people and experiences that I felt overwhelmed. I then devised a drawing exercise: I asked people to make a "map" of their most important relationships at different ages, using circles (Josselson, 1996b). This had wonderful results. People became interested in how to organize their maps (no drawing skill required); then, having created the maps, they were eager to narrate for me which people they placed on the maps and where and why, and they told me very thoughtful and meaningful stories that lay behind their drawings.

Other people have used other forms of visual representation, such as drawings or pictures, to invite narrations. I think of these techniques as "interview aids." They are not measures or standardized in any way; rather, they are means to plunge interviewees into their experiences that relate to the research question and mark a starting point for telling about their lives. Some of these are described in Appendix A.

Most research questions can be addressed with some experience-near little q question to start the conversation. Sometimes participants will respond with a question: "Do you mean . . . ?" or "What do you mean by . . . ?" These are requests for more orientation. You will usually just need to reassure such interviewees that whatever occurred to them to talk about is just fine, but you may need to modify the language of the question so it comes closer to their own life experience.

Big Q (conceptual) question	Recruitment question	Little q (experience–near) question
How do men construct the work–family balance? [Conceptual framework: Male identity.]	I am doing a study of how men manage their work and family responsibilities, and I'd like to talk to you about how this works in your life.	I'd like you to tell me about your work and your family. We can start with either one.
How do girls who have been sexually abused experience telling about their abuse? [Conceptual framework: Secondary trauma in disclosure.]	I want to talk to the girls in this center about what it was like to first tell someone about what happened to you, about how you decided who to tell, and then about what that was like.	Who was the first person you told about what happened, and what do you remember about that?

(cont.)

Big Q (conceptual) question	Recruitment question	Little q (experience-near) question
How do people diagnosed with bipolar disorder manage the way this disorder is socially constructed? [Conceptual framework: Social construction of psychopathology.]	I want to learn about what happens to people when they are first given a diagnosis of bipolar disorder, and what then happens over time.	Please tell me about when you were given a diagnosis of bipolar disorder and how you reacted to this.
How do people with borderline personality disorder experience the therapeutic relationship? [Conceptual framework: Relational structures in borderline personality.]	I am studying people who have been diagnosed with borderline personality disorder and their experiences with psychotherapy.	I'd like to hear about your experiences with your therapists. Please start with whichever one seems most important. (But this question was not put forth until after talking through a good deal of life history material, including what led to the diagnosis.)
How do married women who discover lesbian attractions in adulthood rework their sexual identity? How is sexuality in women "fluid"? [Conceptual framework: Sexual identity and erotic plasticity in women.]	I'm talking to women who discover in adulthood that they are lesbians about what this discovery was like, what they did, and how this led them to think differently about their lives and perhaps make changes.	Please tell me about how you first discovered that you were attracted to a woman, and how this affected you.

Big Q (conceptual) question	Recruitment question	Little q (experience-near) question
How do young people who have lost a parent maintain a continuing bond with their dead parent? [Conceptual framework: The dynamics of grief.]	I am studying people who have lost a parent before they are 18, in order to understand the impact of this experience on their lives.	Please tell me about the parent you lost, when this happened, and something about how and when you have continued to think about your parent ever since.

Launching the Interview with the Little q Question

The novice qualitative researcher, poised to begin an interview, has usually already formed some ideas of what the participant will tell about his or her experiences; these ideas are usually based on the researcher's own experience. This is especially true when the researcher is also a member of the group he or she wishes to study (e.g., immigrants, lesbian/gay/bisexual/transgender [LGBT] people, crime survivors, etc.). I think it is important for researchers to *be participants in their own studies at the outset.* Get someone to interview you (confidentially) with your own question, and *tell your story.* I have found that when researchers have had the opportunity to produce their own stories in great detail, they are less likely to try to "find" those stories in what their participants tell them. They are then more prepared to encounter the fact that others' stories are not what they expect. They are ready to be surprised.

After all the work to prepare an experience-near little q question to launch the interview, a researcher may find that the first discussion is to negotiate a joining of the interviewer's framework and the way the participant thinks about his or her experiential world. The interviewee is trying to match his or her internal representations of experience with what the interviewer seems to want to hear about.

The following is an excerpt from a study on the nature of career satisfaction in CEOs:

> INTERVIEWER: I'd like to hear about the high points of your career . . .
>
> PARTICIPANT: Do you mean times I achieved my goals, or times when I was given awards or promotions—or just times that I was particularly enjoying myself?

The participant's question is meaningful on at least three levels. On the process level, the participant is trying to get straight what kinds of experiences the interviewer wants to hear about. On the content level, there are very interesting data about the participant's having in mind three possible kinds of "high points," so the participant's reframing of the question is itself revealing about the participant's construction of herself and her world. On the relational level, the participant's question may imply a kind of challenge or covert criticism ("You asked me an unclear question"). The best response here, if the interviewer wants to learn about the landscape of career satisfaction, is to say (warmly), "I'd like to hear about all three—in any order." The warmth of the response is meant to be nondefensive, accepting the participant's question and indicating, "It's *your* meanings that interest me." If participants such as this one reshape the initial question, and it is still in the ballpark of the larger research question, the interviewer should try to stay within their construction—because ultimately this is what the interviewer is most interested in exploring. If their narration seems to go far afield of the research interest, the interviewer can always gently guide the focus closer to the primary topic later.

The opening question is meant to direct a participant's attention to his or her own experience (in relation to the little q question) and indicate the interviewer's interest in hearing about that experience. At the process level, the interviewer tries to invite a narration, not an answer. This example is from a recent interview for my longitudinal study of women's identity. I had chosen a very open-ended little q question:

INTERVIEWER (ME): So—I'd like to hear about the last 10 years, since we last talked. What has been most important for you during that time?

PARTICIPANT: Let's see—that would be 1999 . . . I can't remember what was happening in 1999.

ME: It doesn't have to be exact—I mean just this time period, more or less. What has been significant for you?

This interaction is meaningful at the process level. I am signaling that I am not asking an exacting question, that she doesn't have to get it "right." (Her response, of course, reveals something about her need to do things right.) My response invites her to begin anywhere she chooses, and I offer "significant" in place of "important" in hopes that this word will be more engaging as a starting point.

Sometimes our construction of a question is only tangentially relevant to a participant's experience—perhaps because the participant is not a good representative of the population we wish to study, or perhaps because our area of focus is overshadowed by other aspects of a person's life. We can learn from this, but it is often not the kind of understanding we hoped to achieve. I recall one time when I was a participant in a study about fantasies relating to an unborn baby's gender in expecting mothers. A distant acquaintance had recruited me as "a mother willing to talk about experiences during pregnancy." Although my child was by then a teenager, she said that my participation was fine with her, as long as I could remember what I was thinking about while pregnant. I thought it would be a good learning experience for me to participate in a qualitative research interview, and I also wanted to help the researcher out. (My wanting to help is a motive often expressed by participants in qualitative research.) She hadn't mentioned when she recruited me that she was primarily interested in the thoughts or wishes I had in regard to the sex of the unborn baby. (This was fine, from the point of view of the research enterprise, because she hadn't wanted her participants to prepare and package experience before the interview.) So I was surprised when she began by asking me to think back to when I was pregnant and try to remember any thoughts, wishes, or fantasies I had about whether my baby would be a girl or a boy (this was in the days before sophisticated ultrasound). Trying to collaborate, I made an effort to formulate a story of my pregnancy in terms of my thoughts about the sex of my child. But this was difficult. I had a lot of memories about my pregnancy and a lot of awareness of my wishes, conflicts, and anxieties, but only one memory that had anything to do with gender. And that had less to do with gender than with the father of my child. I recall having a sinking feeling at the beginning of this interview, especially since I very much wanted to be cooperative. "I can't make you a gender story," I said, "because gender had so little to do with where I was psychologically with the baby I was carrying. If you want, I can tell you about what was going on, and you can see if you can find gender of the baby as part of it." The researcher agreed, and I don't know what she ended up doing with my interview. The story I told her was, I think, much more superficial than it might have been if I had felt she was interested in the things I actually experienced—things that seemed outside the frame of her attention.

Sometimes we can learn a great deal from people who cannot fit their experience to our formulation. Therefore, the initial negotiation with the participant in which we together try to relate the little q question to the felt realities of personal experience can be very illuminating for the research. If we take as a metaphor life as a weaving, what we are doing with the little q question is asking people to trace a single color through the pattern. Sometimes this will be a dominant color, and it will be easy for them to do. Other times, we discover that what we thought might be a dominant color is actually less so, and in order to trace it, the participant has to give us a broad sense of the whole pattern of the weaving in order to locate and describe the place of the thread that concerns our project.

The little q question is a starting point. The interviewer's response to the opening narration will then determine the course that the interview will take. An interview is something like a chess game, in the sense that the opening can be described in detail, but what happens afterward constitutes the art and the challenge. I return to this point later.

The Other Questions

There is yet another set of questions that you, as a qualitative researcher, must prepare before the first interview. This is the set of auxiliary questions that comprehensively includes what you want to know about the person or the experience under investigation. My colleague Amia Lieblich calls these "pocket questions" because you have them in your pocket if you need them, and just knowing that they are there in your pocket will often make discussion of them appear. Chances are that most of them will be covered in the spontaneous account that the participant gives you, but some areas may be omitted. It is useful to have these questions in mind as the interview proceeds, because they can give you directions to follow from what comes up.

It is helpful to think through how you might phrase some of these questions, especially if they involve possibly emotion-laden or sensitive areas. For example, in my study of women's identity, I may be hearing a life story of unvarying calm and purposeful intention. I have prepared a question to investigate the nether sides of experience that goes something like this: "Most people have something in their life, something like a vice, something that if they think about it they wouldn't necessarily want to do, but they do it anyway. What in your life comes closest to something like this?" These are questions devised for particular kinds of stories that, before the study or in response to other interviews, I realize I'd like to know something about. At the end of the interview, you can review the list of questions and, if anything remains uncovered, you can say, "Something we haven't talked about is, for example, your experiences of friendship over the years. What has this been like for you?" Like your opening question, these should be open-ended and invite stories and exploration. A set of example questions is in Appendix B (taken from my study on identity in women). Of course, once you get to know your interviewee, you may decide that there are some areas that it would be better not to explore, but this consideration is on the plane of the relationship rather than the content.

Do not treat these questions as an interview schedule, though.

Do not ask meaningless questions—that is, questions that would be meaningless to a particular participant—just because they are on the list. Make the questions part of you, so you have a clear sense of what you want to know about, and do glance over them before the end of the interview just in case some important topic has slipped away. At the same time, sometimes looking at the question sheet may legitimize certain questions and make them more palatable to the interviewee, in that questions from the sheet signal that they come from the research enterprise rather than from what might be taken as intrusive idle curiosity. I find that questions about sex and money (the two most sensitive topics) sometimes fall into this category, depending on the interviewee and the kind of relationship we have developed.

The list of questions on your interview guide will evolve as the study proceeds. A narrative study is circular, in the sense that the more you learn about the experiential aspects of your conceptual question, the clearer you will be about what to explore with subsequent participants. One participant, for example, may tell you about how a current relationship with a sister has been important in her life, but you hadn't thought earlier of asking about siblings. You might want to add this to your interview guide list as something to think about during the next interview.

Some IRBs will require that you submit these questions as part of your "interview protocol." They are useful for this purpose in reassuring the IRB about the areas you intend to explore in the interview—as long as you do not get confused into thinking that you are actually going to treat these questions as a protocol.

Length of Interview and Number of Interviews

Most interviews last at least 1 hour, but some may go on for up to 4 hours (with a break or two), depending on whether it is feasible to schedule a second interview in projects that require extensive material. In the planning, it is a good idea to schedule about 2 hours, telling the participant that it is hard to predict just how long it may take to talk through things. You don't want to rush through an interview. If someone has traveled a long distance for the interview, it is best to schedule extra time so that the interview can be completed in one session. If you are located near one another, then it is possible to stop and fix another time to finish. The first interview can continue until someone is tired, and this is more likely to be you. Generally, interviewees get energized with talking and are happy to keep on. But, as the interviewer, you are working hard; paying close attention is strenuous, and there is no point in continuing beyond your endurance.

Depending on your topic and the range of material that you wish to cover, it may be useful to schedule more than one interview. The advantages of a second interview are that you and the participant have gotten to know each other; the participant has had time to reflect on what has already been told; and new material is sure to emerge. The disadvantages of more than one interview are that people are less likely to agree to participate, given the time demands; and sometimes interviewees, having satisfied their curiosity about what the experience is like, drag their feet about scheduling a second interview, and you may be left with partial and therefore unusable material. In my view, perfectly competent qualitative inquiry can be conducted with either single or multiple interview sessions. When setting up the plan to work together, you can tell the participant that you expect to be able to finish in one (or two) meetings, but if it seems that there is still more to cover, you will try to schedule an additional meeting.

You have now done as much preparatory thinking and planning as you can, and you are ready to encounter the interviewee and engage in the process of learning from him or her.

CHAPTER 4

Beginning the Interview

The Place and the Materials

Before you begin the interview, you will have made arrangements for meeting. This should be at a time and place convenient for the participant. The space should be private, in some place where there is a door that you can close. Ideally, this will be an office space, preferably your own. Coffee shops and other public places are not acceptable for maintaining some kind of secure boundary around the conversation. It is permissible to meet in the participant's home, but you should inquire first whether there is a room where you can speak privately. I have had participants offer to meet in their living rooms, where family members wander through. They tell me that it is okay with them if their family members hear what is being said, but this does not create the kind of conditions necessary for a rich and revealing interview. You can simply say that you prefer to conduct the interview in a private space. (Sometimes family members will still peek in, out of curiosity about what is going on. This is okay, as long as they satisfy their curiosity and don't stay.)

It is best to try to arrange the setting with enough space between you for a sense of some distance, but not so much distance as to feel formal or disengaged. You will need some kind of surface between you on which to place your recorder or any questionnaires you may want filled out. A low table is ideal. A desk connotes formality and power relations, and it is best not to have such a large piece of furniture between you. You might also want to leave on this table your list of auxiliary questions, so you can pick it up and refer to it at the end of the interview.

You will need to test your recording equipment before the interview, and it is fine to do this with the interviewee (as long as you have done some preliminary checking beforehand). You want to be sure that your recorder is picking up your interviewee's voice. I always use two recording devices in case one fails. Have extra batteries accessible. I also like to use an external microphone for one of the recorders, but this depends on the quality of your built-in microphone. Put the recording device or microphone on a soft surface like a tablet of paper, which produces a better recording with less static or noise. The aim is to get clear sound that you can transcribe easily.

I use both a cassette recorder and a digital recorder, mainly because I have gotten so accustomed to cassettes over the years. The "down side" of this is that the cassettes need to be turned over and changed, interrupting the interview. The "up side" is that using cassettes calls attention to the recording process; the participant usually forgets that a digital recorder is running continuously, so if there is any discrepancy between what the person is saying "on the record" and "off the record," the digital recorder picks it up. During one long interview where we paused for lunch, the digital recorder picked up the lunchtime conversation—in which I actually learned a great deal about the participant that she didn't think it important to tell me during the more formal interview. Of course, ethics require such material to be treated as "off the record," but it can be useful for understanding context. I am not necessarily recommending this setup, but I do recommend that you use two recording devices in case one fails.

Your Self-Presentation

How you appear will influence the interview. The participant will be reading something about who you are by how you look. The participant will be wondering, "Is this person like me? How does this person fit into my categories of people in the social world?" You can't control participants' perceptions of you, because people will think what they think, and you don't yet know what their social categories may be. But you have to be ready for the possibility that they are misconstruing you. You can control some of the cues you give by how you present yourself. Your gender, race, and age are, of course, immediately apparent and cannot be changed (although age may be misread). What meanings your gender, race, and age (and I include nationality here as well if you speak with a foreign accent) may have to your participants are hard to ascertain at the beginning of the research relationship, but may be revealed as you proceed.

In general, despite all the writing about the various prejudices against women, my experience is that women have an easier time as interviewers than men. Research shows that throughout life, women are more likely to be chosen as confidants than men—by both men and women. Speaking openly to a woman and expecting a nonjudgmental response are more familiar to most people than doing so with a man. Men are often construed as interested in "just the facts." Therefore, men may have to work hard to demonstrate their empathic listening abilities, and may need to be extra careful not to challenge or evaluate. On the other hand, women researchers may have to work to persist in their authority when interviewing men, and may need to resist a tendency to defer to gendered power arrangements. Gender dynamics are most salient when a researcher of one gender is doing research on the world of the other. For example, when a woman is studying war, she can turn the sense of strangeness ("You haven't been there") deftly to her advantage by acknowledging the strangeness and asking for more explanation (Lomsky-Fedder, 1996).

Racial and age differences are sensitive and are likely to be signaled with questions embedded in the narrative about whether the participant's experience could be understood by someone younger or of a different race: "I don't know if you are old enough to remember . . . ," "I don't know if you ever experienced real prejudice . . . ," or the like. The most useful response for the good of the interview is to say lightly, nondefensively, and with some gentle humor if possible, something like this: "Yeah, I had some different experiences from yours, which is in part why I really want to learn about how these things were for you," or "Well, I have been *learning* about how things were [e.g., in the 1960s, in the Deep South, in homeless shelters], but everyone had a somewhat different experience." That is, try to accept rather than camouflage the differences and to use these in the service of asking for explanation. At the moments when, as the interviewer, you feel most aware of difference, remember that the interviewee is the expert and that the point of the interview is to enhance your education and edification. Do not fall prey to an internal sense that you *should* already know something.

Your race, age, and gender are fixed, and you have to deal with whatever assumptions these demographics raise. You can choose what you wear, though, and this will signal something about social relationships. Your dress should make you look serious about your work without being professional in an intimidating way. If you are interviewing business people in their offices, try to look like the kinds of people they are likely to see in their offices. If you are going to someone's home, try to look a bit relaxed without being too casual. If the participant is coming to your office or home, your dress should be professional but comfortable; a suit is probably too formal for this setting.

Similar cautions apply to how you speak. Speech in part signals social class and may also mark educational attainment. As with dress, try to match the parlance of your participants without making yourself ridiculous or unserious. Try not to use any words your participants will not understand; this puts them down. If you are interviewing teenagers and know some of the current slang, you can use it in preference to scholarly language or even in preference to more adult speech if you can do so comfortably.

When you are interviewing people from different cultures or

subcultures, it is a good idea to learn some basic aspects of their history, customs, music, and geography. You certainly don't have to be expert, but it is a good idea to know enough to be able to have a conversation that may refer to places, important historical figures, or holidays, so that the person does not despair of having enough shared knowledge to be able to talk to you. When I was interviewing Ethiopian immigrants to Israel, I tried to learn enough about the different language groups and village areas to be able to ask thoughtfully and understand something about which part of the country people felt was the home they left. Over the course of interviewing a number of people, of course, I learned more about which distinctions were important. On the other hand, I was once interviewing a Finnish participant who had come from Karelia, and I simply had no idea what or where that was. It is a very significant place in Finnish history, especially to its displaced inhabitants. In some ways, my ignorance (which was embarrassing to me) seemed to fit his expectations about Americans. He was quite willing to offer me a brief history lesson so that I could understand his roots and experience better; throughout the rest of the interview, he seemed to try to take care of me by checking to make sure I could keep up when he situated his experience in his larger social world.

Some people have preconceived ideas about academics or about psychologists. These participants will be wondering about why you are interested in *them*, or why you are doing this work at all. It is important to give them some explanation that makes sense to them. Usually, stressing the need for greater understanding of whatever group you are studying is meaningful. You can say something like this: "This is something that we as a field don't know enough about, so I think it important to turn to those who have experienced it to try to reach a better understanding."

Where there are large gaps in social class, such as when academics interview people living in poverty or on the margins of society, participants are likely to feel that they have been objectified and treated as "the Other" by their society. In such cases, they may construe an interview as an opportunity to resist the social definitions of themselves as inferior, but may at the same time present themselves in stereotypical fashion (Krumer-Nevo, 2002). For us as interviewers, our recognition of human complexity must lead us to try to find the whole persons we are interviewing, even when such people seem to fit a two-dimensional societal representation of "the Other." At the same time, we have to be prepared for resistance to express itself in the form of missing interview appointments, being difficult to reach, or other types of nonconformity to what we consider expectable standards of arranging to talk together.

The First Moments

In conducting an interview, we are doing something that is unique and unfamiliar—to both us and our participants. The underlying relational dynamic that has to be acknowledged in some way is this:

> Indeed, this is an unfamiliar situation. You perhaps have never talked to a stranger this way before, and I have never talked to you before. So we are both feeling our way, in hopes that I will learn something of value from you and that it will be meaningful to you to share your experiences with me. I recognize that there may be some bumps as we figure out together how to have this conversation. I will direct the conversation to the areas that are of most interest to me, but most of the time I will try my best just to be with you as you talk to me.

I am not suggesting that you say this out loud, but it might be well to say this to yourself as a way of getting into a frame of mind to begin.

In first meeting a participant, the interviewer must behave in some socially predictable ways. This is why some initial small talk feels "comfortable." It is meant to signal, "We are just two people who can have an ordinary social conversation (even though our plan is to have a different kind of conversation).” During the interview itself, it may sometimes be necessary to revert to ordinary social engagement in the service of this “comfort,” to keep up the conversational flow rather than to establish a more formal interrogatory stance. At the same time, the art of interviewing involves tolerating some discomfort and distinguishing between discomfort as a signal of something awry in the relationship and a signal of something significant or possibly painful emerging in memory and in the narration.

On first meeting, some small talk serves to break the ice, especially if it establishes some kind of commonality, much as it does on a first meeting in a social situation. You want to establish yourself as friendly and warm. It’s fine, if you are meeting in the participant’s home or office, to admire something impersonal (e.g., “What a lovely room” if you think it is, or “What an interesting picture” if you think it is). This suggests that you are curious about the participant, taking in expressions of him- or herself and prepared to respond positively. Try to get a reading of how the participant is initially viewing you. Who do you think the participant thinks you are? And then try to counter any projections you think are there. Answer any questions the participant might ask you about yourself under the cloak of this small talk.

In situations where you are interviewing someone who is likely to “look up” to academics, try to lead with your least intimidating manner, bringing yourself as close to “persons just like you” as possible. I often find that when people know that I am a psychologist and that I have written books, this leads them to treat me like a dignitary to whom they have to be subservient. This is not a good frame for beginning an interview. In such cases, I make a show about dealing with my technology—getting the recorders and microphones tested and working, and making quite genuine comments about my anxiety and uncertainty with these machines. In a sense, I am calling attention to my least competent aspects. This gives participants an opportunity to observe me before I ask them to tell me anything, and I hope it dispels any idea that I know everything or am somehow “above” them. I always accept tea if offered.

The First Interaction

Although as the researcher you have been forming a relationship with each participant from the time of the first thought to work together, the first interaction that is not small talk sets the tone for the interview. It is important to present yourself as serious in purpose, but in a friendly and comfortable way. Seriousness and formality are different, especially when people assume that an interview will be a structured list of questions. You can communicate your seriousness of purpose by describing who you are, for what reason you are doing the study, who is funding it (if there is funding), and what usefulness you expect the overall study to have—and it is best to do this in a straightforward, warm, and conversational tone. In the recruitment conversation, you have told the participant what the interview will entail: "I'll be asking you to tell me about your experiences with [the topic of interest], and the interview will take about an hour and a half. We can meet at a time and place that's convenient for you. Of course, the interview will be completely confidential, and only [my supervisor and] I will ever see the transcripts of the interview." Too often, my students have been intimidated by their institutional review boards (IRBs); in their worry about saying exactly what they told the IRBs they would say, they sound rote, formal, and off-putting. In the first contact, you have to get into a relationship with the participant. This may mean putting your supervisor and IRB further back in your mind as you communicate to the potential participant who you are, what you are doing, and what you will expect of the participant (and where and when). Everything else can be dealt with in later conversations. If you start too formally, then you are in effect inviting the most public, packaged part of your participant to the interview. If you are too informal, you are inviting a chat rather than an interview, but this is usually less of a problem.

As the interview begins and progresses, with its focus on understanding the participant's experience, the participant will become less interested in who the interviewer is beyond how the participant "feels" the empathic response. The interviewer sometimes finds this even more difficult than being pelted with suspicious questions, because the interviewee seems no longer interested in him or her. The interviewer's inner prompting may be to respond with some version of "Me, too" or in some way to share the conversational focus. It takes a lot of practice for an interviewer to stay grounded in his or her interest in the other person.

Formal Consent

At some point in the process before your interview, probably even before a pilot interview, you will have submitted a proposal to your institution's IRB. These committees are increasingly formalistic and formulaic about informed consent, and this is a very bad way to begin an interview. It is, however, necessary. The only way to deal with this necessity is to try to separate the formal aspects of consent from the relationship you are trying to build with the interviewee. Try to soften the consent process as much as possible by linking yourself to it and keeping a distance from it at the same time. Use words that are comfortable for you. I say something like this:

> Before we do anything, I have to introduce a formality. As you may know, before we can do any research at my university [or hospital], we have to have formal informed consent from those who participate in our research. So I have a form that is mandated by my university that I need to ask you to sign. It's kind of long, but what it says basically is that you consent to be interviewed, that you understand that whatever you tell me will be kept completely confidential, that whatever I write about this conversation will disguise your identity so that no one will be able to identify you, and—most important—that you can stop talking to me at any point if you wish to stop.

The participant then looks over the form and signs. (A sample consent form is provided in Appendix C.) You should be prepared to answer any concerns that the participant may have about the form, and make sure that he or she understands its fundamental assurances. Then I say, "Okay, so now we can get on with the interview," hoping that this signals a move to more spontaneity and less distancing formality.

Orienting the Participant to the Question

Begin by reminding the participant about how you have come together: "As you know [or as we discussed on the phone], I am studying [for example] how people who have been chronically ill cope with their illness." Repeat here whatever your recruitment question is. It is best to do this in a conversational way and be ready to talk about your intentions until the participant seems to understand. Then you are at the crucial moment of the interview, for you are about to make a transition between your concerns as a researcher and the participant's experiences. You are, so to speak, passing the "talking stick" to him or her.

Once you feel that your participant understands your research question, lead smoothly into your little q question as a way to orient the participant to what specifically about his or her experience you are interested in hearing about, for example: "So please tell me about [the experience of interest] from the beginning—when did it start, how did you manage, how did things change over time? Tell me whatever you can about how it was for you." I recommend speaking the little q question in as inquiring a way as possible. I try not to sound formal or even very fluent. The question should paint a kind of border around the field of experience you want to know about; it should be an invitation rather than a *question*. It should invite association and exploration rather than an "answer." The aim is to engender a conversation, to make an opening to begin. Exactly how you phrase the question may vary a bit for each interviewee as you find words that seem most suitable for the person you are talking to. It is important for the question not to sound too packaged or formal; try to maintain a conversational tone that will invite a free-flowing response.

However open-ended your initial orienting question may be, what you will hear first is what Labov and Waletzky (1967) call the "orientation." The participant is likely to respond with a relatively short summary—a bottom-line answer, so to speak. Your response to this will be very important. You must follow the summary with interest and a clear indication that you want to hear a lot more detail about the stories and memories that underlie the summary. So your first response should indicate both acceptance and appreciation for the outline, and an interest in having the digest "unpacked." You signal that you want the participant to make a short story long rather than a long story short.

The question in the participant's mind for the first minutes of the interview is "Am I telling you what you want to hear?" There are thousands of ways to narrate one's experience, and the interviewee wants to be sure that he or she is not wasting your time, but is narrating in a way that can be useful to you. (Most people do not want to be telling you a long story when what you really wanted was a short one; this engenders shame.) Your responses to the first narrations shape and define the field of inquiry—the points where your research interest intersects with your participant's lived experience. You signal these points of intersection by what you choose to notice and respond to.

The first responses from the participant will be organized to align themselves with your interest, and also to test out how you will respond to what he or she tells you. These first exchanges are like trying to dance with a new partner. If you respond to what is first offered with another, seemingly unrelated question, then you are implicitly structuring the interview as a question-and-answer exchange in which you lead and the participant follows. If you respond with acceptance and interest, however, you are signaling that you intend to follow the interviewee's lead.

The movement over the course of an interview is from surface to depth, public to private, or thin to thick, depending on which metaphor makes most sense to you. People will begin with their most public, surface faces, painting a thin sketch of their experiences. You want to invite deeper, more private, thicker description of these experiences, and you will do this through your empathic, accepting, nonjudgmental listening.

Sometimes people will offer you a whole road map as a summary, including many aspects of their experience; in effect, they are inviting you to choose which avenue to pursue. You will, of course, want to go down all of these roads, but you have to do so one at a time. So as not to determine the flow, you have several choices about what you will ask a participant to elaborate: You can choose what came first, what came last, or what you think the participant will be most comfortable talking about first. As a general rule, you want to save the more sensitive, emotional aspects of experience for later in the interview, when you have built up more trust together. But you have to make a mental note to go back to these areas, lest the participant think that you are indicating that you are afraid to hear about these experiences. You can always say, at an appropriate moment, "You know, earlier you mentioned [e.g., that during this time you had an abortion], and I wonder if you can tell me more about this and how it affected you."

Once the interview is underway, the interviewer's role is to actively listen, to invite elaboration and detailed stories, and to stay in the relational dance. His or her task is to be an empathic listener, listening from a stance of curiosity and engagement. The interviewer has to be alert for any disruptions in this fundamental relational patterning, and to address them as they occur to get the conversation back on course.

Listening/Responding Stances

The best interviews have the fewest questions. Note that the initial little q question is not really a question, but an orienting inquiry describing the sorts of experiences we as researchers would like our participants to tell us about. A question directs attention in a specific direction—and, if what we are interested in is the structure and organization of the participants' inner world, we want *them* to be doing the painting (to return to an earlier metaphor) without our suggesting what they put into it. A qualitative interview that can be analyzed thematically and deeply requires that the language, the linkages, and the associations belong to the interviewee and not the researcher. Otherwise, the interview becomes a kind of survey, orally administered, and is suitable only for aggregation and coding. Many interviewees may be expecting to have questions put to them sequentially, but most will quickly warm to a different style of inquiry.

What is the problem with asking a question? What happened when I asked you that question? It directed your attention. In order to answer, you had to frame your mind around my question and try to think about problems with questions. Any question in the interview situation takes control and directs—or may even overpower—the process. Sometimes you may want to do that, but you have to do it judiciously and recognize that you have done it.

In order to continue to deepen and extend interview material, we have to be in a listening stance that creates safety and denotes interest. I do not like the word "probe" in this context, because it conjures for me intrusion, penetration, and an absence of mutuality. I prefer to think in terms of exploration. Following an interviewee is also not about "digging," but about requesting elaboration and greater understanding. We can simply think of ourselves as "asking more about" or "extending."

The interviewing stance that will produce the richest narrations is one of *listening*. Listening is active, not passive. We can think of ourselves as actively listening people into speech. As interviewers, we try to maintain a stance of attentive, empathic, nonjudgmental listening in order to invite, even to engender, talk.

In daily life, when we listen to people talking to us, we are generally listening prepared to react from our own experiences, wishes, and set of opinions. In interviewing, the aim is to listen from *inside* the other person—a skill that can be practiced and mastered. In our minds should always be the question "How was this for you?" Of course, the interview will produce a great deal of interesting material that we will want to think about and react to in terms of our own associations, but there will be time for this during the analysis phase. When we have participants before us, we want to use as much time as possible to listen to *their* experience.

Silence

The least intrusive behavior to fulfill this aim is *silence*, sometimes punctuated with assenting sounds such as "Mmm-hmm," or with an affirming smile and nod or a commiserating groan. Silences should not be too long or too short. Generally, novice interviewers err by making silences too short, speaking out of their anxiety that the silence is "making the participant uncomfortable." We want to indicate that we are willing to sit for a moment and think and wait for the next thought to emerge. The idea here is to respond in a way that encourages further thinking and talking. Ideally, the participant will just continue when he or she sees that you are listening and thinking. Indeed, in the silence, you should be thinking about what the participant has just said, never thinking about "What should I ask next?" If your thoughts have gone to "What should I ask next?", then you are attending to your own anxiety rather than listening. In a crunch, you might simply say, "I'm thinking about what you just told me, and I wonder if you can say more about [whatever caught your attention]." As novice interviewers gain experience, they become more comfortable with silence and use the silence to try to picture in their own minds what an interviewee is narrating.

Generally, when novices listen to the recordings of their interviews, they find that what felt to them like a very long silence in which they were afraid they needed to *say* something was actually only a few seconds. If an interviewee remains silent, you can also ask, "Were you having some other thoughts about that?" Such a comment indicates that thinking is also part of the process.

Clarification

A second level of response from the interviewer asks for various forms of *clarification*.

GETTING THE STORY STRAIGHT

Clarification may involve just getting straight what is being told. This is tricky, because you need to be able to understand enough of what someone is telling you to make sense out of it without turning the interview into a question-and-answer dialogue. Most really experienced interviewers ask for clarifications in a somewhat different tone of voice, as though these are "footnotes" to the main story. Clarification questions are relationally complex, because you really want to understand the participant but also don't want to interrupt. If someone mentions a name, a place, or a movie that you are unfamiliar with, then it is important to ask about what the reference is, in order to indicate that you are really trying to follow what the person is communicating. But timing is crucial here, since you don't want to sidetrack the main point by asking for clarification of details. For example, a participant may say, "I felt just like the character in *The Big C.*" But you may not know what that is. So, at a reasonable point (don't interrupt), you might say something like this: "I understand you felt something in common with the character in *The Big C*, but I'm afraid I don't know that show, so could you please tell me a bit about it and what felt similar?"

Clarification questions can be useful at the beginning of an interview for orientation and elucidation of what is offered at the outset. But be careful not to establish a pattern of asking and answering. Questions at the beginning should follow up on the "synopsis" offered by the interviewee, and should be asked only if necessary to show that you are trying to orient to the story (e.g., "When did this happen? How old were you then?"). They should also be kept to a minimum. The focus has to be placed from the beginning on the interviewee's felt experience and their personal story. To some extent, you, as the interviewer, are coming into the middle of a program in progress. You can ask about what you need to know to make sense; the rest you have to try to pick up from context. On the one hand, you don't want to pepper your interview with a lot of questions that interrupt the flow; on the other hand, you don't want to get back to your workspace and have a lot of important references that you don't understand. You need to find the balance, and generally clarification about details can be saved for later unless you are getting lost in the narrative.

Some interviewers who are anxious about getting the chronology right keep asking, "What year was this? When was that?" But doing so interrupts the story. People generally narrate life experiences in a postmodern way, jumping around in time. In such cases, it is best to make a mental note, finish listening to the narration, and then go back at the end of the interview to clarify chronology.

The mind associates things that go together. You may not be clear about what links the associations, but you want the associative process to happen. You can puzzle out later what the links may be; this is part of your interpretive work. If you interrupt the narrative flow too much, you miss out on the associations. If you intervene with a question that changes the subject, you cannot reason that this is a connection within the participant. Rather, it is something you have introduced, and this muddies the waters considerably.

DETAILING THE STORY

Another type of request for clarification is to invite a story that will offer more detail. This is a very useful interview prompt. The request may take the form of "Tell me about a time when this happened," or "Tell me about the last time this happened," or "Can you tell me an example?" This technique can be used when the participant is talking about experience in more general terms or when empathic responses do not elicit elaboration. Here is an example from a study of decisions to change jobs.

JOSH: My boss doesn't trust my judgment. She is always micro-managing me or criticizing me.

INTERVIEWER: She's looking over your shoulder rather than letting you manage things.

Empathic response.

JOSH: Yeah.

INTERVIEWER: That must be difficult for you.

Another empathic response.

JOSH: Yeah.

INTERVIEWER: Could you tell me about a specific incident where this happened?

Clarification—request for a story.

JOSH: It happens every day.

INTERVIEWER: Then tell me about yesterday. What was a time when you felt her micromanaging or criticism?

JOSH: [Responds with a story about his interactions with his boss in a struggle they had yesterday.]

This kind of request for a story will open a shared understanding of what Josh considers micromanaging or criticism, and will also provide a window into important interactions he has in his work environment. Notice, too, that the interviewer is indicating that she really, really wants a story and will not be satisfied with a generality. This will influence the rest of the interview, as Josh now anticipates that the interviewer wants to hear about the specifics of his experience.

MEANINGS

Another kind of listening stance for clarification reflects the meanings the interviewer has understood so far and invites correction and/or elaboration. That is, it summarizes and invites further reflection. It takes the form of (for example) "So if I've understood you, you feel that your boss views you particularly as untrustworthy, for reasons you can't make any sense out of." The interviewee will respond either to affirm ("Yes, it makes no sense at all to me") or to extend ("Well, there are some reasons . . . ").

Clarification of meanings is an effort to try to align the interviewer's developing understandings with the inner world of the participant and generally leads to elaborations. In the excerpt that follows, Megan, a participant in my study of women's identity, had been talking about her struggles with her son, Harry, and I was trying to understand what the struggles were about. Note that my effort to clarify led to a whole different story:

MEGAN: He, he had, uh, he had been involved in a car wreck event. And someone had hit him, and he got some settlement money. And bought himself a cheap car and got a little part-time job. And made just enough money to put gas in it, and that was it.

Here I am not sure how Harry's getting himself a car was related to all the struggles she had been describing with him. I phrase my effort to clarify in a slightly questioning tone.

INTERVIEWER (ME): And that was a source of a lot of tension, strife, arguing . . . ?

MEGAN: Yes, yes . . . yes . . . Oh, I would try and talk to him all the time. I would try and keep him with us, you know, not physically. And one day Harry came home and he started packing his belongings, and he was gonna move out. And that was when it hit Lenny that Harry was leaving, and, and . . . Lenny said, "I don't want ya to go, Harry." And he sat there and he said, "Well I wanna get a few things straight: I don't wanna go to church any more . . ." Now we had never been the kind of parents to say, "You have to go to church. You don't have a choice."

I still don't understand how the car figured in the struggle, but with the new story, I begin to grasp that issues about Harry's independence and autonomy were underlying their struggles. I choose not to return to the car story here, because I think I have caught the drift of Megan's meanings. The car signified Harry's capacity to leave home.

Clarification of meanings can also lead to corrections, where the participant edits or reframes the interviewer's understanding. Here is a participant in my identity study talking about her regular attendance at church:

INTERVIEWER (ME): So you've gone back to your religion . . .

CHARLENE: Um, it's not about religion. I go to my church sometime if it's, like, a family thing. But really when I go to my church again, sometimes I go and I think, well, I'll go again, because the music—all in minor keys, absolutely sad, so sad and so open to heart, so yearning. So the church, they do the incense, it's absolutely beautiful music, but really, I'm not interested in God or . . . I guess, to me, to live a soulful life is to try to be aware, to see the deeper meaning of something, to try to be genuine, authentic, to try to be with people in a way that makes sense to me, but it's not about God.

Note in this excerpt that my comment was aimed to extend Charlene's discussion of church attendance, and my bringing up religion invited her to clarify the meanings I might be making and replace them with her own. Charlene corrected me and offered me a clearer (and quite poetic) portrayal of her spiritual identity. Corrections are extremely valuable efforts to clarify meanings. Experienced interviewers welcome them and do not take them as criticisms. (Occasionally we might say lightly, "Sorry, I misunderstood," but this is rarely necessary.) Sometimes a participant will disown words an interviewer brings into the interview: "I wouldn't say I was *angry* . . . I felt a lot of things, maybe a little annoyance, but mainly frustrated." These are important opportunities to learn about the structure of the interviewee's world.

Empathic Response

The most potent of listening stances is *empathic response*. In this form of response, you as the interviewer empathically experience what has been told, and then reflect your understanding of what the participant has communicated. That is, you try to mirror both the emotional part of the story and the content part of the story. The emotion is what drives the story line, and you must indicate that you resonate with this, or you will encourage a recitation of facts with no life in them. Empathic responses signal that you are understanding ("getting") what is being told, and this understanding becomes a motivating force for the participant to continue. This kind of response sounds straightforward, but it takes a lot of practice. It is so central to good interviewing that it deserves its own chapter.

An empathic response becomes another solution in the moments of silence if you start to get anxious about the silence. Instead of thinking, "What should I say next?", you might simply repeat some aspect of the last narration to indicate that you are empathically thinking about it. If you are clearly focused on getting into empathic contact with what the interviewee is saying, there shouldn't be *awkward* pauses—although there may be *reflective* pauses. Empathy dispels any awkwardness there may be in silence.

Confrontation

Confrontation involves asking the interviewee a challenging question as a way of evoking a justification for something he or she has said or done. It may be done gently, as a way of finding the boundaries of what a participant is describing and thus of understanding more fully. In the following example, the interviewer uses a mild kind of challenge as a way of better locating the interviewee's feelings about her experience.

This excerpt is from a study of personal relationships in high-functioning people diagnosed with borderline personality disorder. The researcher was asking participants to describe interactions with a sequence of people, including strangers. The interviewer's first response in this excerpt was a very empathic reflection of what the participant was describing, and he followed it up by taking one side of the participant's ambivalence to understand better what happens:

> APRIL: Once we were in California, and my husband bought so many local fruits and we didn't know what to do, so I was like, "Oh, I can give it to the beggar." But some of this fruit, according to Chinese medicine, is not good for you. You know, like, the plum, they say, is bad for your system. So I felt, "Maybe I should just throw it away." Anyway, I was carrying this bag and I guess I think I'm doing something good, because I have to go out of my way to look for a homeless person and it's not like I knew where they are. So I'm carrying this huge bag, but I really want to give this to somebody. So I'm looking around, in the meantime feeling like I'm doing something good and maybe also something bad. Like, am I just trying to feel good about myself doing harm? I was thinking about that. Then I saw this guy sitting there, so I put out one thing and asked him, "Is this something you like?" And he nodded. And then I pulled out another one, he nodded. Basically everything, he nodded. So I just gave him the whole bag. And he was like, "Thank you, thank you," and I don't know why, I cried. Maybe because I felt like I helped someone, also maybe like I'm doing something bad. What will happen to his stomach? So I just walked away. I didn't know, I felt, it affects me a lot.

> INTERVIEWER: It was a very poignant moment, but kind of a mixed feeling.

> APRIL: Yeah, maybe I was being too critical. Partly also because I didn't want my husband to eat that, because he doesn't have a good stomach, so I didn't want him to eat all of that. So I felt like I was giving something bad away.

> INTERVIEWER: But for someone who does not have anything to eat . . .

This is the confrontation. Tone of voice is very important here. The tone has to indicate, "I'm interested in better understanding your thinking," and in no way to suggest, "That's a ridiculous idea."

APRIL: I don't know if that's necessarily good. But, yeah, I know, I know, in general it is something good. But I don't understand—I overthink, but I still don't understand why I feel so emotional.

In this excerpt, the interviewer was taking the position that the participant's action seemed to him to have been more of a good gesture than a bad one, raising the question of how it could be bad to offer food to a hungry person. Notice that this led to some distress in April ("yeah, I know, I know"). She felt misunderstood, but offered the observation that "I overthink," which could be an important self-observation to follow. In any case, the interviewer learned from the interaction that there were moments in her relationships, even with strangers, that April felt she didn't understand the emotions that arose and couldn't decide whether what she was doing was good, bad, or both. Moreover, the researcher obtained an excellent example of one such moment and learned about how April responded to other points of view. The interviewer's mild confrontation invited April to further detail her thinking without evoking (too much) shame or defensiveness.

Confrontation, disputation, or argument should be used in interviews very sparingly and carefully, if at all. I once provided consultation to a researcher studying women who had been abused by their partners; she was asking them rather pointedly to justify going back to their violent partners, and then arguing with them quite deliberately and contentiously about what she saw as their "excuses." I suppose that one could thus learn about how such women respond to being challenged in this way, but I think that confrontation invokes defensiveness, and that such an interviewer is likely to close off rather than open up the exploration. I also think that such techniques are ethically dubious. If confrontation is used, there must be a good reason for it, and an interviewer should proceed very cautiously.

Michal Krumer-Nevo (2012) presents an interview from a study of women in poverty, in which she explored through confrontation her interviewees' reasoning (see Krumer-Nevo & Sidi, 2012, pp. 303–304). The interviewee, Sarit, was talking about wanting to be a giving mother in contrast to her own mother, who she felt was depriving.

> SARIT: God gave me these children, and now I live only for them [a short silence]. This is what gives me the strength, makes me want to go on . . . and go to work, and take care of them. At least I have someone to take care of, . . . and I won't make the same mistake as those who took care of me. I . . . I will be everything opposite from what my mom was . . . I will do everything for my children. *Everything.* Whatever . . . I don't know what, there's nothing that I won't do for them, that they never lack anything.

> INTERVIEWER (MICHAL): And what do you think you need to do so that their lives are not like yours was?

> SARIT: I need to . . . first of all, to go out to work, to provide for them . . . but mind you . . . if I get into a situation that I'm working and it doesn't help, the wages from my work, I am capable of stealing, too, and I don't know what I won't do, but they will lack nothing, *nothing* I will let them lack . . . . Whatever they want. Everything, everything, even if it's unnecessary things, whatever they want I'll give them [short silence]. I know that . . . my eldest girl, every time she says to me, "Mommy, chocolate; Mommy, this; Mommy, that," I know it ruins their teeth and I know it's not healthy, but I give her *everything*, the whole day she's on sweets, *the whole day.*

> MICHAL: Really?

> SARIT: . . . I don't want her to be told what I used to be told . . . I grew up on this word, "No, I don't have, and no, I can't give you."

> MICHAL: You know, I understand what you are saying and how much you don't want them to hear these words, "No,

I can't give you," but still . . . I'll ask you a hard question. You know that when she eats chocolate and sweets the whole day, it's bad for her teeth, or when you say, "I'm prepared to steal so that they don't lack anything," it will harm them too. That is, if you steal and go to jail, that's not good for them, or if you get into trouble, it's not good for them; who will take care of them? And if their teeth rot, it's not . . . it's just trouble for years and years. . . .

SARIT: I know, you're right, but it hurts me, it hurts, even if . . . she'll say, "Give me chocolate," and I'll get her some, and then she'll say again, "Give me chocolate." I can't, I don't want to say to her, "No," or "I don't want to give you." Sometimes I say, "You can't have that," and . . . she cries; I see her crying, I'll go and get her all the chocolate there is. Why, when I was little, I would see kids hanging around with sweets, and I would be dying for some sweet, once a year they'd [Sarit's parents] buy for me. I don't want them [Sarit's children] to be like me, I want it to be just the other way around, that other kids are jealous of them. That's what I want, the opposite of what I was.

In her last intervention, Michal gently asked Sarit how she weighed the potential harm in her giving. She prefaced it by saying that she was going to ask a "hard" question, thus signaling that the question would be outside the empathic frame she had established. This kind of confrontation explored the boundaries of Sarit's thinking and had to be raised in an artful way that would not imply judgment or criticism.

Moving Together: The Empathic Attitude

The ideal listening stance is *moving together*. You hope that your interviewee will be moving along the track of your question (i.e., moving with you) at the same time that you are moving along the track of what is important to the interviewee (i.e., moving with him or her). At moments, this may be seamless, a joint motion of interest and disclosure.

Your stance as the researcher/interviewer is to be holding firmly to two ropes: one the rope of the conceptual question (what you, as the researcher, are doing the interview for), and the other the rope of engagement with the participant—the human relationship in which the interview unfolds. If there are moments where your handholds on the ropes feel tenuous or in danger, *always* let go of the conceptual question rope and hold on to the rope of your relationship with the interviewee. In other words, your role as interviewer has to take precedence over your role as researcher. Keep the interview setting as secure as possible, affirm your interest in the interviewee's experience, keep your compassion and concern foregrounded, and follow where the interviewee goes. You can always go back later and pick up the conceptual question rope. If you make the other choice and lose the interviewee by interrupting, criticizing, backing away emotionally, or implying that what he or she is telling you is off track, your interview will turn to dust, and you will be left holding on to your question but no interviewee.

When we are moving together with our interviewees, we are "with" them, following their lead while they are following the lead of our interest in them, tracking one another harmoniously so that the material unfolds seamlessly. We together enter a separate space— not an ordinary conversation, but a place of what Buber (1958) calls "meeting" in a knowledge of another person and an awareness in the other person of having been known. Amia Lieblich (personal communication) contributes another metaphor, that of "walking together on a dark road where I hold the light and walk along with you." Exercise 2 on the facing page provides a sense of how intricate this process of moving together—Buber's "meeting"—is.

The path to moving together is through empathy. I turn in the next chapter to a detailed focus on how to assume an empathic stance and what sorts of verbal responses this entails.

Exercise 2. Moving Together

Do the following exercise with a partner. Ask a third person to time the exercise for 5 minutes (or set a timer clock). This is a nonverbal exercise in which you and your partner stand with your right feet aligned and together, your right hands up at shoulder height, and the palms and fingers of your right hands touching. Close your eyes. You may move all parts of your bodies, but your right feet (which are touching) have to stay together and fixed on the floor. You may move your right arms, but your hands must stay together. Neither of you may talk or make sounds. When the exercise begins, you may begin to move. Notice who seems to be leading and who seems to be following; how this may change over the time allotted; and in particular when you can't tell who is leading and who is following, because it seems that you are just moving together. Take note of the "moving together" feeling, because this is what you hope to achieve in your interviewing skills. Most people who do this exercise feel something profound—and feel a sense of having been in a special dance together.

After the exercise, talk with your partner about what you each experienced. Try to locate moments in which you felt yourselves "moving together," checking to see whether this was mutually experienced.

CHAPTER 5

The Empathic Attitude
of Listening

The aim of a narrative research interview is to enter the world of the participant and try to understand how it looks and feels from the participant's point of view. This occurs through empathic listening. Empathy is a cognitive phenomenon (taking the perspective of another) as well as an affective one (vicariously feeling another's inner experience) (Kerem, Fishman, & Josselson, 2001). We reach an empathic attitude through highly attuned, focused, careful, attentive listening.

Listening is difficult, and understanding is even more so.[1] Good listening means exposing ourselves to the unknown; it involves giving up our usual frameworks and immersing ourselves, intellectually and affectively, in the viewpoints and experiences of the Other. To understand takes a great deal of patience and work—work that demands attention to both the content and emotional tone of what we seek to understand. The challenge to understanding results from there being so many levels to hear and to grapple with; things are both said and unsaid. Meanings are both transparent and hidden. The description of experience always includes both the "facts" (as

---

[1]See Orange (2011), Greenspan (2010), and Andrews (2007).

the participant knows them) and the indicators of how the meanings of those "facts" are to be assessed. Embedded in every narrative is what Labov and Waletzky (1967) call the "evaluation"—the markers of what the experiences meant to the person. These meanings are generally the focus of our studies.

Our default position is not understanding. The less we think we know, the more we are likely to investigate. The participant before us is an unknown individual whom we approach with benign curiosity and a readiness to learn about how this person has been going about life. We are poised to be open to and accepting of whatever we might hear. We expect to be surprised and to grapple (together) with indeterminate meanings; we recognize that things will not be "clear." If we imagine ourselves as trying to get "answers" to our "questions," we have moved outside the dance of creating shared understanding. At the end of the interview, we may feel enlightened, but the indeterminacy will remain. (We will make further sense of the material during the analysis.)

Our orientation to what is transpiring in the conversation will be affected by nonverbal exchanges as well as by what is said. We will be either consciously or subliminally aware of when the participant moves away from us, shifts uncomfortably in the chair, makes eye contact to search for a response from us or looks off in the distance, fidgets, smiles, or brightens. None of this will be on the audio recording, so if we can keep track of it, we include these observations in the notes we make after the interview. Beyond noting these instances, however, if we are empathically attuned, we will be responding as we listen, and we may be able to hear in our own voices in the recording our empathic attunement to the emotional state of the interviewee—matching joy, sadness, fear, guilt, outrage, worry, contentment, or pride.

Empathic listening demands focused attunement and is very hard work. Most people take for granted that they are skilled at listening, but few really are. In everyday life, we listen very partially—taking in bits of the sound that we hear and meshing these bits with our own thoughts, which actually claim more of our attention. The act of artful listening involves clearing out our mental houses for a time and opening our minds and hearts to what is coming in. It is an act of un-self-consciousness, of becoming something like a mirror. (Indeed, the neuroscientists tell us that the parts of our brains that are active when we are empathically attuned are the "mirror neurons.") We must stay fully in the present moment, undistracted by the outside world or by what we might say next. When we attune successfully, the interview becomes a very gratifying experience for the participant, who feels truly heard. In my workshops, I ask, "When was the last time someone just sat and listened to you for 2 hours?" Usually my students just laugh in response to this question. None can recall such an experience. In social life, we take turns in conversations; we express ourselves in short bursts of speech. We don't expect that people will have enough interest in us to pay sustained attention just to us. This is why many participants in interview studies feel that the opportunity to speak about themselves has been integrative or healing for them. All we have to do as interviewers is to listen well.

Empathic Responsiveness

The aim of the interviewer, then, is to move with the interviewee, doing verbally as well as nonverbally what happens in the "moving together" exercise (see Exercise 2 at the end of Chapter 4). This requires empathically attuning to the feelings that are connected with the events being narrated, demonstrating to the participant that the interviewer is mentally capable of putting oneself in his or her place (Bourdieu & Wacquant, 1992). This is, of course, first an internal response—a necessary first response before the interviewer makes a verbal response. To be fully empathic, the interviewer must allow him- or herself to be emotionally touched, to resonate with the experience being narrated. At the same time, at the level of thought, the interviewer must ask him- or herself, "What have I understood from the interviewee's communication? What is the interviewee's point of view?"

The listener's understanding will be increased by more specific detail—the stories of lived experience, rather than generalities about a life. It is important, then, to communicate interest in the actual instances of what the participant is describing, and the interviewer may prompt with "Tell me about a time that happened," or "When was the first/last time you remember this happening?" in order to direct attention to actual stories. It is in recounting the specific aspects of an experience that the interviewee's experience will become fully present in the interview and the interviewer will be able to be "right there" with the interviewee.

Working from this internal understanding, the interviewer might then offer one of the following verbal responses (if something beyond silence or acknowledgment seems necessary for maintaining the conversation):

1. *Summarizing.* This kind of intervention takes the form of "So what I've understood from what you said is that you . . ." This is a way of noting that you have been hearing what the participant has been saying, and the summary will invite either acknowledgment ("Yes, that's right"), correction ("Well, it wasn't exactly like that"), or further detail. Summarizing is a way for you to clarify meaning by asking, "This is what I got. Did I get it right?" Summarizing carefully stays with the same words that the interviewee chose. A summary will often invite further discourse, but a simple "Right" or "Yes" from the interviewee is a signal for you to choose the next direction—either to request other examples, or to pick up something else from the earlier narration or from another aspect of your interview plan.

2. *Paraphrasing.* This is related to summarizing, but it condenses the account or focuses on some essence of particular interest to you as a researcher. You may gingerly and cautiously introduce some new words into the interchange to determine whether they "fit" the participant's experience. If paraphrasing is empathic, it will lead to further elaboration. Examples:

"So this was a kind of epiphany for you," or "So it seems like this was a time you kind of hit bottom."

3. *Mirroring.* This involves reflection of feeling. This response expressively focuses on the feelings communicated in the account and invites elaboration on the emotional level. It has the form of "So you were feeling _____ when that happened." The participant may not have named the feeling, but you have detected it from the tone of voice or facial expression, and in your response you lightly, tentatively name it. In other words, you try to match the feeling, not declare it.

In general, beyond getting the main plot of the story the participant wants to tell (what happened), following the feelings in the account will open deeper and more complex layers of experience. Empathy is both cognitive and affective. You must be able both to know and to feel with the interviewee. If the interview takes the affective route, there will be richer lodes of meaning, because what will be expressed is how the events being recounted had an impact on and became significant to the participant. The parts of the story where the interviewee felt joyful, excited, proud, moved, sad, disappointed, envious, guilty, angry, or resentful are the points of greatest arousal, and thus central to how he or she accounts for whatever changes or experiences are at the center of the research question. A good mirroring response conveys that you have understood the participant at the level of feelings being expressed, without in any way distorting the content.

Strong feelings indicate that something important is lodged in this part of the story and should entice rather than repel you. One of your primary tasks as the interviewer is what Bion (1962) calls "containment"—holding, absorbing, and staying present with feelings. It has the sense of "I can feel this with you," without having to get rid of the feeling. You just need to stay with the feeling while the participant shepherds it into words and follow it wherever it goes. If you flee from affect, the message this sends to the participant is to stay on the surface, at a distance from what was experienced.

Probably the most frequent question I hear in workshops is about what to do if a participant cries. The students who raise this question are perhaps worried about feeling embarrassed and "not knowing what to do." There is no "doing" that is required. An interviewer can simply sit quietly and wait for the participant to gather him- or herself and continue speaking. Listening empathically, the interviewer tries to convey an understanding of what the incident being described felt like to the participant. The interviewer might say gently, "I see you have strong feelings about this" or try to reflect the nature of the feeling and see where the participant takes the narration.

In rare cases, and I mean really rare, where the participant seems too upset to continue (see Good Interview 3 in Chapter 7), you might suggest going on to something else and perhaps coming back to this later. You have to use your empathy and sensitivity here. You might ask the participant whether he or she wishes to go to something else if you aren't sure. If the participant apologizes for tears, it is important to say that no apology is necessary: "Of course people feel strongly when talking about difficult or painful things." This normalizes what is, after all, quite normal.

Once a student told me quite sheepishly, with great shame and trepidation, that during an interview in which her interviewee grew tearful while talking about the sudden death of her mother, she got tearful as well, and tears streamed down her face. My student expected me, it seems, to chastise her and tell her she had lost her role (and no doubt wasn't suited for this kind of work). Instead, I commented that it seems that she was indeed in empathic attunement to her participant.

So often, students I am supervising will tell me that they were interested in some difficult aspect of a participant's life, but the participant "didn't want to talk about it." When we look more closely, it is usually the students who became skittish about the area and backed away by changing the subject.[2] So who is it, I wonder, who

---

[2] See Hollway and Jefferson (2000) for elaboration of the idea of the "defended researcher."

didn't want to talk about it? Some students are afraid of "making people talk about things they don't want to talk about." In general, participants are in control of themselves and what they tell you. There is no way to *make* participants in a research interview tell what they don't want to tell. It may be true, however, that in a relationship with an empathic, accepting listener, people will tell more than they had expected they would. In such cases, there is no coercion, only invitation and opportunity.

Some people have asked me whether it is okay to laugh with participants if they tell funny stories that they laugh at themselves. Of course it is fine to do this. The principle is to match the participants' feeling—and to try not to inject your own.

Emotional expression is not unitary. People often have more than one feeling about an event, and the aim is to try to empathize with all the feelings that are being expressed. The most common interviewer error here is to "hear" just one feeling state and follow that—usually the one that makes most sense to an interviewer, the one the interviewer thinks he or she would have been most likely to have experienced in that situation, leaving aside the other feelings. This will result in a skewed view of the experience at the interpretation phase. Here is an example. This segment is from a study about reactions to loss and processes of grieving; the interviewee and participant were women of similar age.

> PARTICIPANT: It was a terrible blow when my boyfriend broke up with me, but all my friends gathered around me, and I realized that there were a lot of people who cared for me, and they helped me move on and apply to graduate school. I realized how many resources I had and how much good there was in my life.

> INTERVIEWER: So you forged ahead, feeling that you had a lot of love and potential in your life.

A better response would be this: "So you forged ahead, feeling you had a lot of love and potential in your life, but it had been a terrible blow." This response would pick up both sides of the emotional experience and leave the interviewee free to elaborate either side of it. The interviewer must be interested in hearing about the complex interplay of experience, not just a simple story line. The interviewer could, of course, return to the other side of this experience later. The mistake would be to recognize only one aspect of the affect—in this case, to privilege the happy ending over the "blow."

Empathic Questions

Although I have said previously that the ideal empathic response is a reflection rather than a question, and that this is a skill you should practice, in actuality interviewers do ask questions. It is possible to phrase a question empathically, picking up an element from the previous narrative passage and asking for elaboration. Such questions take the form of "What was that like for you?", "Tell me more about what you meant by that," or "How did that feel to you?"

A question beginning with "Why . . ." usually has accusatory or judgmental overtones, and it is better to expunge this word from your vocabulary. If you want to know why someone did something, ask, "What sorts of things were in your mind when you chose that course of action?" or "How did that come about?"

An empathic question follows the flow of the narration by inviting the next part of the story. Or it might ask for amplification of a part of the story that was told cursorily or just referenced obliquely. As with reflections, you need to be paying attention to the feelings being expressed in the course of the narration and following the affect. Strong feelings point to aspects of experience that were meaningful to the participant, and these moments should be noted and inquired into. Sometimes only a question will do, even if it's in the form of "You mentioned this difficult time in your life. Can you tell me more about that?" Empathic questions should seem to the interviewee to be designed for him or her and to derive from their experience, rather than to be prepackaged or taken off of a list.

Here is an excerpt from an interview study of adult women

who had lived as heterosexuals and become lesbians in adulthood.[3] This excerpt begins with good empathic responses, but then goes off track:

> SOPHIE: You know, you're looked at differently. I can remember, early on in our relationship, going out, and I had kind of the, I was very aware of being looked at in public because of who I was with. When you're straight, you don't worry about that. Nobody looks twice at you. And, um, you know, again, I was a person who wasn't used to getting a lot of attention. And all of a sudden I feel like I have this attention on me. And, again, you know, to be labeled something that is stigmatizing, and you know you're going to lose certain things . . . your rights. [Laughs, then suddenly becomes serious.] You know, that was really scary. My partner's always known and she grew up, you know, being kind of different because she is Polynesian and, and, and, 'cause she is lesbian too. So I kind of had a real hard time probably for about 2 years, adopting that, you know, that label.

> INTERVIEWER: You mentioned stigma a couple times and having a hard time "adopting the label."

> *Note that this excellent response falls in between a reflection and a question. It is a reflection that invites elaboration, rooted in what Sophie has been talking about. It concerns a central aspect of the researcher's Big Q question, but is asked unobtrusively within the flow of the interview, linked to the participant's experience as it was emerging in her memory.*

> SOPHIE: In the beginning it was not good. I . . . [long hesitation] I was drinking [face turned to the side, voice lowered]. A lot. In the beginning. Gosh, I'm trying to think. That was not a good period of time. The first three years were really tough. I spent a lot of money, um, that's how I was coping. I spent *a lot* of money. I put myself into massive debt. So, and then, I finally was like, "Okay, I have got to, I, I, I, I know I have the genetic makeup to be an

---

[3]This study was conducted by Jeanne Miller for her dissertation.

alcoholic, so I gotta quit this stuff." And you know, I had to just, kind of . . . I remember one day sitting down and just going, "I gotta get my life on track, I gotta get my stuff in order," you know? My partner and I weren't doing well at the time because she's not a drinker, and I was literally going to, you gotta remember too, I grew up so sheltered and in such a strict family, I went right from my parents' house to my husband's house and I never, I never had that. You know, that kids have that adolescence, you know, that young adults go through, kind of out having fun.

So it was the first time that I was really doing anything like that. It was the first time, you know, that I had this group of friends, um, who I was hanging out with. And they were all kind of drinkers. And they didn't have any coping skills, so I kind of adopted what they were doing. So when I got away from them because, I remember thinking, "I gotta get away from them, these people here, gotta get away," you know, because I just felt like I was not being who I was.

That's pretty much how I coped back then. I was part of this group; it was a generalized support group open to LGBT, that's no longer being run, and it kind of turned into a free-for-all. There was really no structure. I felt like it was a place for people to get together, and the guys were all hooking up together, and the girls were trying to hook up together.

INTERVIEWER: Is that the group you were going out with?

This is a side clarification, and the participant goes on.

SOPHIE: Yeah, I was hanging out with that group. Now I do have two very good friends from the group that I totally exclude from, but most of them were really toxic people to be around. They just didn't have healthy lifestyles. They were doing lots of drinking. And again, I grew up, so, for me to put myself in that . . . Now I can't stand to be around someone who has a drink. And that's really, truly who I am, I just kind of stay away from that. So to just kind of submerge myself in that, you know, I just wasn't myself.

And my girlfriend, who never had a drink in her whole life, she probably had a big hand in getting me out of that, because I knew she was not going to stick around if I continued on the path, so yeah.

INTERVIEWER: So that's how you came out of that, you made some decisions and she was there . . .

This is a fine reflection of what has come last, but it ignores the obviously difficult but important material about the period of the participant's being out of control—a period that coincided with her coming out, so it is important for understanding in the context of the research question. It may be a good choice, though, to wait to see whether Sophie spontaneously picks up that part of her story.

SOPHIE: I did. I remember her saying, "I'm worried about you, you're doing these things, and you know, you're kind of being self-destructive." And I remember sitting down, and thinking to myself, "All right, I gotta get my life in order." I am very organized, I mean, I make lists for everything. I do. I remember I sat down one day, and I made a list of this is stuff that I need to do to get my life back on track, and I started knocking them out.

Sophie's narrative here had many intertwined elements and presented a challenge to the interviewer. Empathically, the interviewer recognized that coming out, stigma, being out of control, drinking and spending and the evolving relationship with her lesbian partner were all interconnected. Sophie seemed to be saying that her partner was the catalyst for getting her life under control, but this was not clear. What was especially unclear was whether "accepting the label" of being a lesbian initiated or resolved the "out of control" period. The challenge here was to find an empathic response that would hold all of these elements while they were still emotionally close. The breaks in Sophie's speech indicated that there was emotional pain connected to memories of this period, so the interviewer would need to move gently. One possible intervention would be this:

So you got your life back on track (*acknowledging the good outcome*). I wonder, though, (*signaling a shift in the other direction*) if you would tell me more about that difficult period you had. It sounds like your drinking and spending and coming out all kind of happened together (*asking about the overlap among these experiences rather than trying to bring the feelings themselves to the surface, which would be more of a therapeutic avenue*). And somehow stigma was part of the whole thing (*to try to understand the links in the progression of the interviewee's thoughts from stigma to the out-of-control period, to the influence of her partner.*)

Empathy and the Big Q Question

The more of an expert you become about your research question and the themes that you want to investigate, the more you will be able to empathically engage your participant in helping you to learn about these themes in the participant's particular life. In this way, you can find and enlarge the themes of interest to you as you empathically attend to what the participant tells you. It then becomes unnecessary to pose a direct question. When the participant is talking about something close to "what you really want to know about," you will perk up internally and pursue that avenue with an empathic lead. For example, in a study about felt relationships to teachers at school in relation to academic success, the researcher began by asking about best and worst experiences at school:

> PARTICIPANT: Junior year was the worst. My friends kind of snubbed me and I didn't like my classes. I was doing okay gradewise, except in history, but that teacher didn't like me.

> INTERVIEWER: You thought that teacher didn't like you . . .

If the study were about friendships or academic preferences, the interviewer would have empathically followed these elements of the narration instead of the relationship with the teacher, which was the focus of the researcher's interest.

Using Empathy to Follow the Story

Questions can empathically follow the story, picking out the most salient meanings and asking further about them. These kinds of questions are voiced in the same tone as the respondent is using, thus empathically matching the feelings that are being expressed. Empathic questions differ from questions that redirect or change the course of the interview. Note the differences in the excerpt below, which is from my study of identity development in women. This participant had been somewhat difficult to interview, because she mainly narrated other people's stories and talked about herself only in brief generalities. She was clearly uncomfortable with self-disclosure, but she had spoken about having a crisis in her marriage and going with her husband to couple therapy.

> INTERVIEWER (ME): What has your experience of therapy been like?

A very open-ended question.

> ZELDA: Yeah. She's sort of helping me, you know, realize . . . that I tend to be . . . I tend to be fairly rigid about things and see things in my own particular way, and there is more than one way to do it, and how Frank sees things is not necessarily how I see things. Uh, so that's . . . [looking at me expectantly]

> ME: Can you think of an example?

Noting all the hesitance in the speech here, I invite a story rather than pursuing "rigid" (another option), especially in light of how guarded this interviewee has been.

> ZELDA: [Long pause] . . . This is a pretty simple one. Frank

was going to buy a car, and I feel pretty strongly that I hate noise, and he was originally going to get an alarm in his car, and . . . we talked about it, but for some reason, I had this feeling that he didn't necessarily hear what I was saying, 'cause . . . so I asked him to repeat, you know, what I wanted as far as the car goes. And it took a bit, but it was clear that he definitely hadn't heard what my concerns were, and before I actually would . . . it would not have occurred to me to do that, and basically I'd be fairly explicit without getting excited and understand that just because you see something one way, that's not necessarily how it is or how other people perceive it. I don't know if that's helpful.

ME: So this was news to you about yourself?

I am picking up the change aspects of this story and empathically restate the sense of learning something new about herself, especially in that I am unclear about what she had learned. In linking her example to the question, I am implicitly indicating that the story is indeed "helpful." I am also careful not to take any kind of judgmental position on her change or how she used to be. "News to you" is as neutral as I can be and still empathically highlight the sense of learning about herself.

ZELDA: Yeah. I know I tend to be fairly rigid.

ME: What does "rigid" mean for you?

*She comes back to "rigid" and is perhaps ready to discuss this aspect of herself. Note that in picking up her word and asking her to expand it, I am trying to make clear what **her** meanings are. It is always a good idea to recognize that people have their own definitions of words, and we cannot assume that they are using words the same way we are. This is especially true when there are sociocultural differences, but also true in general. It is best to inquire about words that appear to be loaded with meanings.*

ZELDA: Um, like, I could remember from when I was a kid, I think it was in the May procession from school, and I was the person who was leading it, and there was a very set way we were supposed to go around the church. And the priest went one way and he went the wrong way, so I went the other. [Laughs.] It probably would have been better to just follow and do it the way he went, even though it wasn't the right one. So . . . And probably with accounting [her profession], it serves me well that I tend to be obsessive–compulsive and pay attention to details, but in relationships, it's not the best thing to do.

Inviting this elaboration leads to new and important material. She expands the idea of "rigid" to include a focus on doing it right, even if this means challenging authority. Also, we see Zelda spontaneously commenting on the positive side of her "rigidity," which includes her professionally useful attention to detail. If the study had some particular interest in issues of authority or autonomy, I could at this point follow the thread of "going one's own way in the interest of what is right." I could also follow the idea of learning that what works professionally does not serve her well in relationships and ask for other examples. Such choices are made depending on the overall aim of a study and the material a researcher hopes to obtain and analyze. In this instance, given that my project is about identity development, I decide to pick up the thread of the story the participant is telling about how she has learned something new about herself and changed.

ME: So what you did differently was ask him to repeat what he heard so you could check.

I am summarizing the main point of the "how I changed" story, in hopes of picking up and deepening this topic.

ZELDA: Yeah. It wouldn't have occurred to me. He would have gone off and got the alarm, and I would have gotten angry.

ME: So the old scenario was: You say what your concerns are, he didn't hear you, did what he wanted, and then you'd feel your concerns were overlooked.

I am summarizing in hopes of further elaboration and reflection.

ZELDA: Right, and that's something that happened a number of times. We clearly were not communicating. He wasn't hearing, and I thought I was being very explicit, but clearly not from his mindset.

ME: So this is one way the therapist has been helpful to you—to help you make your feelings very explicit.

I am summarizing and reflecting her meanings.

ZELDA: Yeah, and even if it's something I very much want. I'm trying to think of an example. I think it was—Frank came back from a business trip and said he was thinking of buying a company he used to work for and was unhappy working there. And I said, "If that's something you want to do, you can, but I under no circumstances want to have the house mortgaged to pay for it. If you're going to do it, you need to arrange financing without the house being at issue." He wasn't, you know, happy with that, but I also felt really strongly that I've been working hard to get the mortgage paid off and to do something and he not be happy with it, um, you know, that that would not be a good thing. So . . . he sort of dropped it.

ME: And do you think you would have handled that differently in the past?

I have many choices for response here. The participant ends her narration with "So . . . he sort of dropped it." Both the pause after "So" and the "sort of" indicate that there is a great deal more to this story. But this is a participant who has spent much of the interview largely talking about her husband, his family, and his choices, and the research question is about changes in her identity over time. Thus I am trying to keep her narration centered as much as possible on her experience of herself. In this segment, the discussion is focused on the question of how she feels she has changed, so this follow-up question pursues that direction.

ZELDA: I might have been inclined to think that if that's something he wanted to do, then we should work at it and try to do it, while I would have been really unhappy. So it's given me not permission, but . . . to protect myself and take care of myself as far as what feels reasonable for me.

I now feel that I have an understanding of the theme of getting more explicit about communicating her wishes. The participant has developed the theme, with stories, of having moved from supporting what her hus-

band wanted even if it made her angry or unhappy to learning to speak
her own views. I could ask for an example from the past in which she
went along with something and was "really unhappy," but I feel I have
enough understanding of this theme to proceed. I am also afraid of land-
ing back into another long story about Frank, of which I have already
heard many. I note that in this last narration, Zelda has opened up a
lot and spontaneously offered an example, perhaps because she is feeling
that I am hearing her meanings. So I return to the main question and
invite another theme.

ME: What has been another important thing you have learned
about yourself or about life in the last 10 years?

Personal Reactions and the Empathic Attitude

Our stance as interviewers of maintaining an empathic attitude
means keeping our personal reactions to the material out of the
interview. This can be difficult when participants have views or
experiences that we are in fact quite judgmental about. One of the
people I interviewed for a study on relationships talked of the closeness he felt to his buddies when they went yearly to Alaska to shoot
bears. This was difficult for me to listen to. One of my favorite movies is *The Bear*, a movie about an orphaned bear cub and a wounded
giant grizzly and their efforts to protect themselves from hunters.
I was quite horrified by listening to how they bonded over killing
bears. Similarly, when a participant in my women's identity study,
in describing her political views, vehemently advocated that the
United States should "nuke the Arab terrorists," I found it a challenge to contain my repulsion. In both instances, I had to keep my
(strong) reactions to myself and try to stay focused on understanding
how my participants had come to these positions. If, however, my
participants had nevertheless picked up my response, I would have
acknowledged my difference, apologized, and declared that I was
nevertheless still interested in understanding their experiences and
views.

Just as we are not there to judge our participants critically, we are also not there to praise or reassure them. If we respond to something a participant says with "I think that's wonderful," then it understandably raises a question in the interviewee's mind when we do not respond in the same way to something else. We can acknowledge achievements by saying, "It sounds like you are very proud of this," or "What a sense of accomplishment you must have had," thus staying in an empathic stance, reflecting on the person's experience of their deeds or honors rather than our own judgment of them. A resonant "Wow!" to someone who tells of a great success in an excited way is sufficiently ambiguous to be acceptable; it is then empathic rather than complimentary. Containment implies hearing, acknowledging, accepting, extending, and wanting to understand more. Judgments, good or bad, change the atmosphere and the dynamics of the research relationship.

Sometimes interviewees imagine that we are experts on mental health or moral living and invite our opinions, even asking directly, "What do you think of what I did?" At such times, I often respond by generalizing and normalizing, saying something like "So many people, more than you imagine, have experienced something similar," or "You know, as a psychologist I know that there is no right way to handle this." One of my interviewees disclosed to me that she had been sexually abused as a child by her (now deceased) grandfather, and that her therapist urged her to confront him with this, but that she refused and left therapy. She then began debating with herself about whether she had done the right thing, clearly inviting me into this debate (she knew I was also a therapist). This was, I thought, one of those times where telling her (feelingly) that I believe that there is not a "right" way, that all choices have their benefits and costs, was the best response I could make. In part, I was responding to the unspoken question about whether I was just like her therapist, so my comment had the underlying message that I was a different person—and that I was trying to understand her rather than tell her what to do. My response did seem to reassure her enough that she could continue with her narration.

Empathy and Identification

Another personal reaction that is sometimes useful to furthering the interview and sometimes intrusive is identification. Identification involves finding something in one's own experience that seems to match what the participant is narrating. At such times, one is tempted to say, "Me, too." This can further the interview if the interviewee seems to be doubting that the interviewer could possibly understand, but it can also detract from the interviewee's sense that the interviewer is trying to understand the uniqueness of the participant's experience.

In a study of women who joined the Occupy Wall Street protests, one of my students, Julia, was interviewing a woman living on welfare. The woman described herself as the mother of twin daughters, age 2. As it happened, Julia also had twin daughters, age 3, but (appropriately) resisted the temptation to say so when her participant first mentioned this. Later in the interview, the following exchange occurred:

PARTICIPANT (RICKI): I have these twin daughters. They are just 2. And they always need their diapers changed at the same time. Or one wakes up in the night and wakes the other one, and I have two who are crying. You can't imagine how hard it is!

INTERVIEWER (JULIA): Actually, I have twin daughters myself, so I know something about how hard it is [with a smile, very empathically].

RICKI: Do you have a husband?

JULIA: Yes.

RICKI: Then you can't imagine what it's like to do this all alone.

*Julia's response has been offered in a spirit of empathy, but Ricki makes clear that Julia's experience could not be anything like **her** experience.*

JULIA: Yes, I can imagine that taking care of twins all alone would be much more difficult, very difficult indeed. Please tell me about how you have managed.

In this last response, the interviewer returns to a fully empathic stance.

Empathy always involves some internal identification, a capacity to resonate with and therefore understand, but leaving a space for difference. Identification on its own does not constitute an empathic response and may impede understanding the other person as other.

"Bumps in the Road" of Empathy

As I have said at the beginning of this chapter, maintaining an empathic stance is difficult. There will always be "bumps in the road." The essence of the stance is "Help me understand this so I can be there with you." But the other person is just that—other; that is, different from you. If it seems really easy, then you are likely to be identifying with your participant rather than empathizing, projecting yourself into the participant rather than encountering an *other* person. The process of an interview is one of continually getting in contact, losing the contact, and regaining it. Sometimes, though, interviewees will just close the door on an aspect of their lives—perhaps something they don't really understand in themselves or are unwilling to talk about, despite our best efforts at gentle invitation. At these times we just have to move on gracefully. (Grace in this context means never giving the interviewees the impression that they are letting you down or not "giving you what you want.") Exercises 3 and 4 on pages 100 and 101 are designed to give you practice with getting in contact and maintaining it for longer periods.

The possibilities for empathy are influenced by the dynamics of the relationship and how it is structured, situated, and experienced by the participant. You can expect to be "tested" by the participant, especially at the beginning of the interview. The participant is "test-

Exercise 3. Interview Practice: All Empathy, No Questions

The task is to interview without asking any questions. Arrange a 15-minute interview with a colleague or classmate on a topic of your choice. Begin by orienting your interviewee to the question you want to explore, and then try to respond throughout the interview with empathic responses that invite elaboration rather than with questions. Record your interview and then listen to it later, noting the places where you got stuck and felt you *had* to ask a question. In this review, try to think about how you could have inquired without a question. This exercise will help in decreasing your reliance on questions to propel the interview. Repeat this exercise until you can do it relatively smoothly.

ing" how well (and in what areas) you can truly "move with" him or her. This process is, of course, influenced by who the interviewee thinks you are, how you have framed the research in relation to the participant, and the other dynamics of the relationship that I have discussed in Chapter 2. In the next chapter, I return to, and provide a wider view of, the research relationship.

Exercise 4. Round-Robin Interviewing

We rarely get meaningful feedback from our interviewees, and this makes it difficult to notice how we ourselves might get in the way of creating an engaging interview. This exercise is designed to produce such feedback and can be repeated. It is best to do this exercise with at least five people, so that no two people interview each other. Going down the line, each person interviews in turn two people for 15 minutes with the same question. No one interviews someone who has interviewed him or her. (If there are five people, A interviews B and C; B interviews C and D; C interviews D and E; D interviews A and E; E interviews A and B. Two of these interviews can be taking place simultaneously, with the fifth person writing feedback to be given later to his or her interviewer.)

After the interviews are over, groups of three meet (each group includes an interviewer and the two people he or she has interviewed). Each person who was interviewed by that interviewer offers feedback about how he or she experienced the interviewer's listening. What made the person feel that the interviewer was in contact with him or her? At what points did the person feel out of contact? Were there any moments of feeling judged? What interviewer responses led the person to want to tell more? What responses led him or her to decide not to tell something that came to mind?

Each person has the opportunity to experience the differences in interviewing styles as an interviewee. The contrast in experience helps to sharpen the feedback. The benefit of having feedback from two people who have responded to the same question is that the interviewer can also learn about how he or she can be experienced differently by different people.

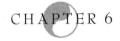

CHAPTER 6

The Research Relationship, Part II

Ethics and Humanity

I have now considered some of the mechanics and techniques of interviewing, and have situated these in the framework of the research relationship that is continually developing. Indeed, as we have seen, whatever is taking place in terms of creating interview data is also taking place at the level of the relationship that is in process. We can only speak about one at a time, but these two levels are co-occurring in an interpenetrating way. What is told is a function of the listener, and the listener is responding to both the felt relationship and the content of the narration. This chapter focuses on the ethics and dynamics of what is taking place in the research relationship.

Topics that are of interest to researchers usually involve aspects of life that challenge people in some way or that arouse conflict, either internal or external. Any good story focuses on some kind of "trouble": It disrupts what is canonical and expectable by detailing what was outside of the ordinary and how a person (or people) responded. Although there are many good stories of happy surprises, many narratives told in qualitative research concern periods of time where a participant was solving some life problem; felt sad, angry, or frustrated; felt thwarted or unjustly treated; or had to cope with great difficulties related to, for example, health, natural disaster, or social injustice. Some investigations focus on problem solving, and there are often strong feelings associated with the problem to be solved. As people talk about these experiences in the personal terms that narrative interviewing invites, human responses from interviewers are necessary. People are, after all, talking about their lives.

Ethics and Interpretations

Although you are doing "research," you are entering a human relationship, and you want your participants to come away with a sense of having been valued. Yet the ethics of narrative research are generally conceived in terms of damage control, of doing no harm, rather than in terms of the ethical value of the opportunity to speak to and be heard by an accepting, attentive other.

If you are listening well, people will open up and speak about very private aspects of their lives—perhaps things they have never told anyone else. As a researcher, then, you have a special responsibility to receive what you are given without tampering with it in any way. Participants may make new meanings about their lives or experiences, or may feel increased understanding of themselves, but you should not offer your own interpretations to the participant. There may, however, be strong temptations to do so, even direct invitations, particularly at the end of the interview as you are packing up and trying to say goodbye. For instance, a participant may ask, "So what do you think? Am I normal?"

This is a baldly stated question, and although it may be camouflaged with different words, it is one that often underlies the questions a participant poses at the end of an interview. The participant has just disclosed very private stories and may worry that there is something unique and strange about him or her. The researcher here *must* respond in a normalizing fashion that says, in effect, "Your experience is shared by others. You are not alone in this. We are both human." My own response to the bald question would be something like this:

> Well, I don't really know what 'normal' is, but I can certainly understand your experience, and I know that others have responded to these life events in similar ways. I also find a lot in common with you. I feel very moved by what you have told me, and I hope I can make what you have told me useful in some ways to others.

If you are at all psychologically minded (and you probably are, or you wouldn't likely be doing this kind of research), you may think you see connections or alternative understandings of your participants' lives that they don't see. Consider this example:

> PARTICIPANT: [She is speaking of her teacher, with whom she had a long affair.] He was a brilliant man, had published a lot of books and had a dazzling wit, and I really tried to get close to him, and I fell in love with him and . . .
>
> INTERVIEWER: It seems like he reminded you of your father.
>
> *The interviewer's interpretation may be accurate, but her response is unwarranted, if not unethical.*

Save such insights for the analysis phase, when you will see whether you can document them from the text of the interview transcript. You may not, however, offer them to the participant. This would constitute an interpretation of his or her life, and that is out of bounds, no matter how clever your interpretation might be. Your aim is to detail your participant's self-understanding, and staying in an empathic stance will keep you from straying from this path.

Humanity

The basic principle of interviewing is that you are human first, and the research relationship is a human relationship. If serious emotional difficulties should occur during the interview, you need to respond in human terms, including doing what you can to lower the emotional temperature and return to less fraught areas. Sometimes simple acceptance is all that a participant requires. Sometimes what the participant needs is for you to be fully present as a fellow human being, putting aside for the moment your researcher role.

After about 2 hours of an interview with Amy, an unmarried, childless woman in my longitudinal study of identity, I asked her to tell me about her happiest memory. To my great surprise, she blocked on this and couldn't think of one. She became quite upset. I quote the dialogue at some length, because I want to demonstrate the way in which I attended to the relationship and helped her regain emotional control by giving her time and making myself present. This would not have been the only way to do this, but I relied on my own humanity at this moment.

> AMY: [Long pause] . . . Like, I have a hard time remembering them, happy moments.

> INTERVIEWER (ME): Well, you just *store* them differently. I think that everybody stores memory somewhat differently, so it's always hard to find out how to, to find out exactly how to ask the question so that it gets—at that part of the person's memory that—

> *I first try to normalize her blocking and suggest a reason for it, taking the responsibility on myself for asking the question in a way that doesn't fit her experience.*

> AMY: There may be some experiences that people have that are really definite. For instance, you know, like if someone got married—you might say, "That was the happiest day of my life."

ME: Mmm-hmm . . .

AMY: And, um, or, uh, "the day I had my uh, my, uh child,"
you know. [She is beginning to cry.]

ME: I'm not so sure of that. Maybe what they think of is called
"canonical memory," that in a sense people have a sense
that that's what they're supposed to say.

*At this point, I begin to understand that trying to think about happy
memories is plunging Amy into regrets about what she has not had in
life. I try talking to her in a reassuring way, intellectualizing so that she
can perhaps regain some cognitive control. I'm also suggesting to her that
there are other ways in life to be happy, and that she can perhaps locate
other kinds of happy experiences in her memories.*

AMY: Ohhh. [She is still crying.]

ME: So, and, I trust more the—a memory that comes based on
experience—because, you know, it's just like an easy out,
and when you see how hard it is, really, to locate these—

*I am now trying to speak to her experience of the difficulty of locating her
own happy memories, and I am letting her know that I neither expect
nor value a particular kind of memory.*

AMY: . . . Yeah—

ME: —things that are important. So I think that if I ask somebody that and they say, "Oh, the day I got married," I think
it's just so easy to reach for that, this milestone, and like—

AMY: Sure!

*Here Amy seems to be joining me and brightening a little, crying less,
so I am encouraged to continue in this vein. I could suggest we go on
to something else, but I fear that this will leave her feeling even more
ashamed and bereft. I think it important that she find a happy memory
to tell me about in order to help her avoid having a sense of failure here,
so I keep talking.*

ME: —and I would think that most people don't even remember the day they got married. It's like on the day that I got

married, with my first husband—the wedding I had, I don't remember it.

Now I'm babbling a bit, trying to give her time to collect herself and regret less not having a happiest memory of a wedding.

AMY: [Laughs.]

ME: I was just in a fog, you know—

AMY: Yeah.

ME: I was so anxious, and all these people, and all this stuff—

Encouraged by her laughter, I keep on with this. I note that Amy has now begun empathically listening to me!

AMY: Mmm-hmm.

ME: And it wasn't until I got the pictures that I even had a sense of having been there.

AMY: Yeah.

ME: So to me it's one of those things we're *supposed* to remember, that are not—

AMY: Right. Yeah, you're right—our memories are more difficult, but I think it has to do with me, and when I'm thinking about it and maybe a couple of descriptions are, have to be with, having, having like, someone wanting to be with me. And, like, um, you know, like wanting to spend time with me. Like that brings me happiness.

ME: Mmm-hmm.

AMY: So, you know, and being accepted.

ME: Mmm-hmm. And that's not just like one incident, that's just in general . . . ?

Here I feel it is safe to resume my interviewer role, as Amy is calmer, has stopped crying, and has pulled the focus back to herself.

AMY: Sure, when I'm thinking about when I'm most happy, it's usually those kinds of things, and of course it has to be someone that I, you know, want to be with, too. But, um, that's, to me, I think where I've been my most happy, yes.

She reveals something about herself that I think is quite profound.

AMY: And I do have people like that in my life. And, you know, you helped me remember that [laughs], by coming out here. Um, you know, thank you.

My way of dealing with this difficult moment was to use my humanity. There was no "therapy" involved.

An interview can occasion the memory of pain, but it does not induce the pain. The pain that emerges is usually related to memories that have been buried and are likely to get buried again after the interview, perhaps with a bit less sting for having been aired and shared. As the interviewer, you respond by recognizing the pain with some form of "I can see how difficult this has been for you."

In the example with Amy above, I tried to assuage the unexpected distress connected to locating a happy memory by trying to assure her that there was no particular happy memory I expected her to have, and that I did not have a "happy memory" of a wedding day either. My seemingly innocuous question plunged her into a pothole in her psychological organization; it went straight to the core of her regrets about her life. I did not try to reassure her about these regrets, to suggest that she had a happy life anyway, or to offer any other patronizing sort of false uplift or advice. To do any of these would suggest that I had some right to try to alter her feelings about her life, which I did not. I did, however, try to take responsibility for the form of my question over which she tripped into the pothole, and to reframe the question about what constitutes a "happy memory" in a way that she could join more readily.

Difficult emotional moments in interviews generally involve either sadness (from loss or regret) or anger. In general, acknowledging the feeling empathically will be enough to help the participant stay in narrative control. Anger will sometimes lead to overfocus: The participant may spend a great of time detailing a sense of

Exercise 5. Difficult Moments

Choose a partner who is also working on improving interview skills. Think about some interpersonal scenario that you fear could happen in an interview, and then role-play it for about 10 minutes, with your partner in the role of interviewer while you role-play the participant. Then discuss what occurred and in what other ways the interviewer could have responded. After this discussion, role-play the scenario again, switching roles (with your partner now playing the participant and you the interviewer).

mistreatment or injustice with many examples, one after the other. There are moments in such interviews where you may have to say something like "I can see how angry you are at your boss and how many ways he has undercut you," and then redirect the interview to something else. Exercise 5 above may prove very useful in helping you learn to manage these and other difficult moments in interviews.

The Research Relationship in Progress

Unlike psychotherapy, the research relationship is not itself a focus for discussion unless it is hindering a free flow of thoughts and associations in the interview. If this occurs, it is important to discuss the participant's experience of the interview itself as it is occurring. One not uncommon occurrence is for the participant to say at the outset that he or she is "nervous" about being interviewed. You can accept this and ask, "Is there something in particular you are aware of being nervous about?" If this doesn't produce anything specific that you can address, I would suggest telling the participant, "Okay, well, if you still feel nervous after we've talked for a bit, please tell me, and we can see how you are experiencing our conversation." Often the issue is something about "what you think of me." It is then important to say something like this: "I think what you are telling me is very interesting and very helpful to me in learning about people who [restate what your study is about]."

It is also possible that, during the interview, the participant may seem to close down rather than open up. You may see this in shorter responses or in body language. It is important to address this by saying, "I wonder if I said something that may have offended you . . . if so, please tell me what it was." Or you can pause in your focus on content and say to the participant, "I want to check in with you and see how this interview is going for you so far. Does it feel okay to be talking to me about these things?"

One participant I was interviewing seemed to be offering more concise and simplified responses rather than telling me much detail in her narratives, and I asked her about how the interview was going for her:

> PARTICIPANT: I just feel so ordinary. There's nothing very interesting in my life. I'm just like everyone else.
>
> INTERVIEWER (ME): Well, the ordinary, as you put it, is just what I am trying to learn about. Maybe you seem ordinary to yourself, because you live with yourself all the time. But I am very interested in learning about the details of your life and how you make the decisions and choices that you make.

This response reaffirmed my interest in the participant and addressed what she imagined to be my expectations of the material she was offering me. It also, of course, told me something about her views of herself. Note that in this example I chose to respond to the relational issues because I had noticed that her responsiveness was decreasing. Another option would have been to inquire more about her sense of ordinariness (thus addressing the content of what she expressed), but keeping the research relationship intact and collaborative should always take priority.

The Research Relationship and Psychotherapy

Some narrative researchers are also therapists (or wish they were). But there has to be a firm boundary between these roles. In psychotherapy, the patient (client) comes to the therapist for help; in research, the researcher comes to the participant for help. This is the crucial distinction, and as a researcher, you have to get this absolutely clear. It does sometimes happen that if sensitive or painful areas of a person open up in the interview, the participant will look to you for some kind of helpful intervention. As I have discussed above, a human response is ethically necessary, but an effort to make a therapeutic response is ethically suspect. If the pressure from the participant for some kind of therapeutic response is great, you can, at the end of the interview, ask the participant whether therapy is something he or she has thought about pursuing. You can add, "Not that I am recommending it, but you seem to have suggested that there are areas of your life that you wish to talk more about and understand better."

My best example of this comes from a man I interviewed for my relational experiences study, who had told me at the outset that he probably didn't have much to tell me. Four hours later, I was still having a hard time bringing the interview to a close, mainly because he had begun examining a troubled relationship with his brother and accessed a long-forgotten memory that gave him a lot of pain. He wanted to keep talking about it, and each time I tried to tell him that he had been very generous in sharing his life stories and I had quite enough material for my study, he launched into another story about this brother, with great pain just beneath the surface. Finally, I said to him that I saw that this was something he wanted to keep on talking about, that something quite meaningful had opened up for him, and that there were counselors whose job it was to help people sort through such experiences. Would he like me to help him find such a person to talk to? He kept on talking. But having made this suggestion, I returned to it more vigorously: "I can't really help you with this, but I'd be more than happy to help you find someone who *could* help you." Then I had to explain a bit about how therapy works by telling him that I was just there as a researcher learning about the pattern of relationships in people's lives, and he had been very helpful to me in that regard. But unfortunately, I wasn't there to try to help him examine his life in a way that would most benefit him—that's not what research does, but it is what therapy does—and I'd help him find a therapist if he wished. He never followed up on this, though, as far as I know. I didn't think I did him any harm in listening to what emerged for him in this interview. And note that I did not *recommend* therapy for him. I only suggested that therapy is a way to continue to talk and examine one's life or relationships, which he seemed very much to want to do.

The Research Relationship from the Side of the Researcher

Doing narrative interviews has little in common with "collecting data" in a more impersonal study. In narrative interviewing, *you,* as the researcher, are the instrumentation. Listening intensely and emotionally aligning yourself with someone's internal world in order to respond empathically will have profound psychological effects on you. In trying to learn from your participants, you will be inviting them to have an impact on you, to challenge your thinking, to extend your habitual ways of knowing, and to reveal aspects of human experience that may be quite new to you. In a good interview, you will be emotionally as well as cognitively engaged. There will be moments of such intense identification with the participant that you will feel you have lost yourself; there will be moments of such strong flooding by your own memories or associations that you will fear that you have lost contact with your participant. With experience in doing such interviewing, you will largely be able to maintain a balance between your capacity to think about the material being offered and being fully present with the interviewee, noting your own feelings but not being captured by them.

Qualitative research is a much more emotion-laden approach to knowledge than the objectifying stance of quantitative work, which occurs at a great deal more personal distance from those who are being studied. Doing in-depth interviews empathically and relationally arouses strong feelings in researchers. Many have debated the use of this emotional knowledge in the larger discourse, which still privileges objectifying reports. Feminist researchers and those whose work is focused on social justice, in particular, have strongly advocated for the importance of emotional knowledge in scholarly writing (Fine, 1994; Fine, Weis, Wong, & Weseen, 2000; Kitzinger & Wilkinson, 1996; Behar, 1996, 2003; Ellis, 2009; Granek, 2012). Regardless of how researchers intend to use their emotional reactions to their participants in the report, these will occur and will inform their understanding.

Doing this kind of interviewing is very tiring, and it is not a good idea to schedule more than one or two interviews in a day. What is most important is to give yourself time after each interview to write down the thoughts, feelings, and impressions that occurred to you during and after the interview. Do not wait to do this; they fade quickly and can't be recaptured.

After transcribing the recording, it is important to review the interview to supervise the relationship you have created. Early in your experience, it is best to do this with a supervisor/professor. Once you gain some experience, you can work with peer collaborators, and eventually you can supervise yourself.

It is easy to set rules—but harder to put them into practice. I have begun this chapter by emphasizing the importance of treating participants with respect, sensitivity, and tact, and of being accepting and nonjudgmental. So imagine my chagrin when, in reviewing some of my transcripts for this book, I stumbled across one in which I told a participant that she "shouldn't feel that way." In my view, this is a cardinal sin in *any* relationship, and I was astonished to find myself saying this. The context was that the participant was expressing her distress that an old painful experience that she thought she had "put away somewhere" was still with her and would always haunt her. (The best empathic response would have been "It never completely goes away.") In my self-supervision, I could see that what I was trying to do was to enlarge her context; I went on to say (empathically) that this difficult experience had different places in her mind at different times. Still, I wondered, during my review, why I was trying to help her manage her feelings—and what I learned was that she had told me that she often turned to friends for just this purpose. I was also able to see from the transcript how critical she consistently was about her own feelings, repeatedly berating herself for what she felt in her various experiences. So I was able to learn something about her, particularly about her relationships with people, as well as about my poor response to her. I wondered why I was having difficulty containing *her* difficulty containing her feelings. This interchange occurred late in the interview, and we had already established a research relationship. Reading the rest of the interview, I could not see that my comment had much effect. My participant pretty much ignored my remark—perhaps taking it in as a clumsy effort at some kind of reassurance, which it was—and went on. My point here is that although we intend to conduct the relationship with our participants in a particular way, we may not succeed perfectly. It is important to review our lapses, acknowledge them, learn from them, and try to do better the next time.

The Research Relationship and the IRB

These days, approval is needed from an institution's IRB in order to carry out any research project with human subjects. Filling out an IRB form is an opportunity to think through in advance any possible ethical issues that may arise during the research process. Researchers must ethically be able to guarantee confidentiality and anonymity through protection of the recordings and the transcriptions, and through adequate disguise of whatever will be written. Researchers must also make it clear to participants that their participation is *always* voluntary and that they have the right to withdraw from the research at any time. I think that students should also submit letters from their supervisors stating that they are capable of sensitively conducting in-depth interviews; this is something super-visors can determine through review of pilot or practice interviews.

Although IRBs are in place to protect participants, the mem-bers of many IRBs don't really understand qualitative research and imagine that they can and should control every aspect of the process, which is, of course, impossible (Lincoln, 2005; Cannella & Lincoln, 2007; Josselson, 2007). They are accustomed to formalized, well-controlled experiments and are frequently unprepared to evaluate interview plans that are flexible, evolving, exploratory, and interac-tive. Often IRBs are more attuned to protecting their institutions from imagined lawsuits than to thinking seriously about the welfare of the participants and the likely import of the research. Except in very rare instances, talking openly with an interested and sensitive listener is not a dangerous activity. Beginning an interview relation-ship with a lot of cautions and warnings is more likely to frighten participants than to protect them (see also Fine et al., 2000). Cer-tainly, it is important to tell people that they may stop an interview at any time with no repercussions. That is, they can simply quit talking if they become too uncomfortable to want to continue. This has never happened to me, but I expect I could respond graciously if someone were to indicate that he or she wanted to stop talking to me.

A researcher may need to educate the members of an IRB about qualitative research by explaining the process of the interview and the general areas that will be covered. If the IRB asks for particular statements in the consent form, the researcher will need to think about the impact of these statements on the participants and on the interviews that will take place under the shadow of such warn-ings—and the researcher may have to negotiate the requirements. The content of the "informed consent" form mandated by IRBs generally derives from forms appropriate to other disciplines, such as medicine.

Of course, when a researcher is going through the IRB review process, his or her inclination may be to submit to its requirements in order to get the proposal approved. But the researcher must pay very careful attention to what is required in the consent form, because asking a participant to sign this form will be one of the first interactions in the research relationship with each participant. Thus, signing this form unavoidably becomes part of the research relationship and must be carefully managed. It is advisable to try to make the informed consent form as brief and user-friendly as possible (see Appendix C for an example).

One requirement that has sometimes been proposed by the IRB at my own university, and that I have heard about at some other institutions, is that the informed consent form must state that participants who become upset in the interview will be referred for psychotherapy. (This is a statement crafted by overzealous lawyers who have no understanding whatever of interview-based research.) One compromise here is for the researcher to assure the IRB that he or she will keep a list of therapists to whom to refer any participants seeming to need such referrals—but I think the researcher should insist that he or she will not state this on the form participants sign. I think the reasons for this stance are too obvious to detail: What does it mean to warn participants ahead of time that they "might become upset," or that if they do so, the researcher will conclude that they need therapeutic intervention? Such a statement is demeaning, disrespectful, and potentially destructive of the interview enterprise. People do sometimes have strong feelings during an interview, but they recover without therapeutic intervention. Do we want to warn our participants that if they should cry, we will send them to a therapist? There is almost no evidence that people who participate in research interviews ever become distressed enough to require intervention, even trauma survivors or people with previously diagnosed and/or treated mental illness. So a statement (or even an attitude) such as "If you seem upset, I will refer you," is poisonous to the whole enterprise in the service of protecting no one. In my experience, IRBs usually give way on this ill-considered dictate.

As I have said earlier, a researcher should tell participants that the informed consent is required by someone else and is standard practice, but the researcher should emphasize his or her commitment to the protection of confidentiality, stress the safeguards that have been put in place, and remind the participants that they are free to stop the interview at any time. In other words, the researcher makes a personal commitment to an ethical stance, rather than relying on the consent form to do it.

The Research Relationship and the Ethics of the Research

Signing an informed consent form does not solve the many ethical dilemmas of interview-based research (see Josselson, 2007). The ethics of the research relationship go beyond satisfying the requirements of IRBs and are, in some ways, more stringent than these requirements. We have an ongoing ethical duty to protect the privacy and dignity of those whose lives we study (Josselson, 2007). Ethics in narrative research "is not a matter of abstractly correct behavior" (Patai, 1991, p. 145), but of responsibility in human relationships (Clandinin & Connelly, 2000). As researchers, we must maintain an ethical attitude at every moment of the research process and be attuned to the ethical dilemmas that arise.

One of these dilemmas is that people cannot in an informed way give consent to their participation at the outset of the study—although they can give consent to participation in the interview. What a participant will tell you will be affected by your capacity to be empathic, nonjudgmental, concerned, tolerant, and emotionally responsive. The data you obtain will reflect the degree of openness and self-disclosure the participant felt was warranted and appropriate under the *relational* circumstances he or she experienced. The extent of self-disclosure will coincide with the degree of rapport and with growing trust that you will treat the material with respect and compassion. I think that informed consent from an ethical point of view requires asking participants at the *end* of the interview whether they still give their consent for you to use their material in the study. At this point, they know what they have told you and can, if they wish, indicate areas that they might not want you to discuss in your written report. Sometimes, during the course of an interview, a partici-

pant will say, "I don't want you to write about this." If participants
flag areas that they don't want you to write about, you cannot do so,
at least not without further discussion with them. It is possible, as
you are writing up the results, that you will want to use a detailed
analysis of a case where a participant has noted areas that he or she
wants excluded. You can, at this point, arrange a phone conversation
with the participant to discuss a proposal for a disguised version to
appear in your writing—but if the participant still doesn't want the
material used, even under disguised conditions, you cannot use it.

Careful steps must be taken to assure anonymity and protect
confidentiality once the interview is transcribed. Transcripts should
be kept in a locked file without the names of the participants attached.
You should also change proper nouns (other people's names, place
names, company names) that appear in the transcripts, or use just
first letters of these names (but keep in a separate locked file a guide
to what you have done, or you may become hopelessly confused at
a later point). You have to use your judgment here and not become
too obsessive about it, but keep in mind what you would worry
about if someone were to steal or hack into your computer. The
point is that the participants should not be identifiable under any
circumstances.

The research relationship continues through publication. The
issues of what it means to write about other people, particularly
if these persons may read what you have written, are thorny and
complex.[1] They derive from the inherent dual relationship in this
kind of research: You have a relationship to the scholarly community that is the foundation of justification for the study, *and* you have
a very personal, empathic, and human relationship with your participants. When you are with your participants, interviewing them
about private, intimate aspects of their lives, you try to be fully
with them. Afterward, you return to your researcher role: You "use"
their material in the service of understanding your topic, and you
speak to the audience of your scholarly peers *about* them. In most

---

[1]See Josselson (1996c, 2007, 2011) for full discussion of these issues.

cases, you can fully protect the participants' identity, so no one can know whom you are writing about. But if the participants will read what you have written, you are still in continuing conversation with those particular people and have to take care to protect their sense of dignity.

In some cases, if you are doing research on a small community where people might be able to guess at one another's identity, you may need to get permission from all involved participants to publish the material—after they have seen what you have written. If you are a researcher in education, you also have to consider these issues when interviewing multiple people in the same school. The dangers of disrupting community life when one person has said something unflattering about another are great, and you cannot take these risks without consent. There are no hard and fast guidelines here (see Lieblich, 1996). You must be aware of the potential consequences of publication and censor accordingly.

Saying Goodbye

There is usually a great deal of intimacy in a narrative research interview, and both the researcher and the participant feel it. Saying goodbye then becomes an important part of the process. The end of the interview does not erase the prohibitions about making judgments, either good or bad. But as the interviewer, you can speak of having felt moved or touched or enlightened by aspects of a participant's life story, or sad about his or her sorrows. And you must always express gratitude for the participant's open, generous sharing of experience. Before I say goodbye, I always give my interviewees an opening to ask me any questions they may have, and I answer them as honestly as I can. I also ask them about how the interview experience has been for them: "How was it for you to be talking to me in this way?" This question sometimes reveals lingering discomfort about judgments they think I may have been making about them, and it also gives me an opportunity to learn about how the participants have experienced me. I then ask, "What questions do you have for me as we end our time together?"

As a researcher, you need to say goodbye to each participant in human terms. This may mean being willing at the end of the interview to talk a bit about yourself if this would help the participant feel more on an equal footing with you or less exposed. In this final phase, you must say something human and sincere about your experience in the interview, but should reemphasize your role as a researcher: "I appreciate your openness and willingness to share your experiences with me. I feel that I have learned a lot from you that will help me in my work." If you were particularly touched by the interview experience, it is fine to say so and to add that you will remember the participant. This is a time when you can speak from your heart (without overdoing it).

Sometimes a participant wishes to continue the relationship. Especially when you are working with lonely or vulnerable people, the special attention offered in an interview may be so gratifying that the participant wishes for its continuation (Booth, 1999). In such circumstances, you must gently but clearly restate your role as having just a certain amount of time to devote to each participant. With such participants, it is probably better to schedule an interview in a single sitting. Multiple interviews over time are more likely to encourage the fantasy of a continuing relationship.

An ethical, well-structured research relationship, in which the participant is engaged with the research question and with an attuned listener, is the platform for an interview that will inform the research. I turn in the next chapter to what a good interview looks like in practice and what makes a good interview good.

CHAPTER 7

The Good Interview

When I look at an interview transcript, I can usually tell whether it is a good interview at first glance, because the amount of interviewee text vastly overshadows the interviewer's interventions. In the best possible interview, there is primarily narration from the interviewee, interspersed with a few responses from the interviewer. In a poor interview, there is a lot of turn taking, a lot of questions and answers. A good interview also has prompts that invite elaboration or the production of illustrative narratives. This chapter presents some annotated examples of good interviewing technique.

Good Interview 1

The first interview comes from a class exercise. The interviewer had no prior knowledge of the participant's experiences with grief, so he was taking something of a risk here. (In an actual study, participants would be prescreened.) The interviewer is male; the participant, Willa, was female; both were in midlife.

> INTERVIEWER: I'm interested in finding out how people overcome the grief of losing a loved one to death. So could you

please tell me about how you've overcome the grief of losing a loved one through death?

*This is a good orienting (little q) question, although it makes the assump-
tion that grief has been "overcome." Still, this is something that Willa
can modify to describe her own experience more fully.*

WILLA: Okay. Um, well, I think first of all, I haven't had a
lot of deaths. I haven't experienced a lot of deaths. So, um,
I can only say there have been two very close people that
. . . my grandfather and grandmother. Um, and my grandfather, I think I was too young to really understand if I
did feel any grief. Um, with my grandmother too, um, she
was . . . it just happened this September. So she was 92 or
going on 93, and for the last year her health and mental
capacities were really declined. And um, she was brought
to the hospital, so, um, we were told that, right before she
died, a week before she died, we were told that, um, that
she had cancer in her spine. And we knew that she was in
really great pain. So, um, the death in a way was kind of a
relief, um, and um and it's really hard to say exactly how I
dealt with it, because I don't know, because of that relief. It
wasn't a death that came on suddenly. It wasn't a death that
. . . even though I miss her dearly, um, it was very, very
hard. It was very hard. So, um—

INTERVIEWER: So you say you miss her dearly. What are some
of the things you think about or do when you find yourself
missing her?

*The interviewer follows the synopsis Willa has offered by using her last
statement as a springboard to invite elaboration. He signals that he is
interested in the specifics of her experience, and this response also shows
Willa that he is paying attention to what she is saying, rather than following some prepared script.*

WILLA: There are some moments that I, you know, feel so
regretful, you know, because um, at the time, at the time,
you know, I was the person who really had to, um . . . I
was more of the person who was really trying to take care
of her and trying to get her help, and it was very difficult

because she was very independent all of her life, up until last year. So, you know, um, you know I think she was very resentful for that. So there are some times that I'm very regretful, and I wish I could have that time to tell her, you know, "I was thinking of you, and, um, I want to protect you," and I think there's also times that I don't think she really understood who I was. She didn't quite understand why I didn't have children, why I was still going to school. So those were times I would feel regretful. But then there's other times that I'm really thankful for and I miss . . . that I had her for 40-something years of my life, and I treasure that. And she was there when I was growing up, and I miss those experiences with her, I miss being a child with her, and, um, I really miss being a child with her. So, I think you know, I think probably, if I think about it, right after her death . . . One of the things I used to love about my grandmother is she had all of these old photographs of her family and my grandfather's family, um, you know, photographs back in . . . of their grandparents and of her . . . and we don't have a—I have a very small family, I'm an only child, so it's me, my mom, and was my grandmother, and I have two cousins . . . and that's it, basically, um, but we have these old photographs, and, um, so what I did is, my mom just had them scattered everywhere, and so I made these photo albums—of all the old pictures, and that was one thing, you know, I did when she was in her deathbed, just really tried to tell her that that's one thing I really loved doing with her, just looking at old photographs she used to like to show, show everybody, um . . . So I think that's if I . . . if, you know, I really didn't even think about it . . . that's how I dealt with my grief, because I would probably say, yeah, it was a relief. We got to say goodbye, we didn't want her to be in pain any more . . . but, um, it was those photo albums. . . . So you know I had photo albums, and I just put them all together . . . photo albums of, like, her great-grandparents, my grandfather's great-grandparents. Photos like when my grandfather was a police officer in Cincinnati. She was, like, a young waitress . . . she would get all dolled up. I learned so much, so I would, like, review it with my mom—and my mom would tell stories of her childhood, like—and I found out so many things, like they would take driving vacations from Florida, all the way down to Mexico. So I think that that really helped. Just that, you know, really enjoying something that I used to enjoy with her that I hadn't done in a long, long, time . . . because I was taking care of her.

INTERVIEWER: And so that was one way to kind of help you feel better, or overcome the loss that you experienced?

This is an empathic response that invites further elaboration.

WILLA: Yeah, I wouldn't really say "overcome," because you know, um, even though I missed her, I would say we were ready. I mean, I was ready for quite a while, but I would say I got to recapture some of the experiences that I used to love with her, whereas within the last couple of years, our relationship was contentious, because I would say, "Hey, you need someone to help you," and basically I was telling her she's not independent any more. And so, and then, you know, at the very end of having to feed her and help her and, um, worry about her, and so—you know, this reminded me when—times when probably the opposite, you know, she was telling me. And we were sharing the experiences that we both really enjoyed—and we hadn't done that for a very long time. So, um, yeah, it made me appreciate something that I had lost for quite a while. I think that probably helped, and I really appreciated it.

Note that Willa corrects the misaligned empathic response ("I wouldn't really say 'overcome'"), which is very useful for the researcher's purposes. She explains that "overcome" does not fit her emotional experience, and she goes on to tell more about the complexity of her grieving.

INTERVIEWER: Mmm-hmm.

Here the interviewer holds the reflective space open; note that Willa continues.

WILLA: I had some—you know, we laughed, and really enjoyed the experience.

There is much rich material in this short interview, reflecting the empathic skill of the interviewer.

Good Interview 2

Here is an excerpt from a very lengthy interview of a woman participating in a study of long-time lesbians who decide to marry men. The interviewer had established good rapport with this very self-aware woman, Hadley, who had told a detailed and complex story about her loss of her relationship with her lesbian partner and her eventual switch to an involvement with a man—something that she hadn't imagined possible for her. Both interviewer and participant were women in midlife.

HADLEY: That afternoon with Daniel, I felt like there was this energy between us, and I don't know, I'll never know, like, what part came from him and what part came from me. And then he called me and invited me to go to a party with him. We had dinner and then went to this party. And that felt like more of a date to me, because it was an evening thing.

So we went to this party. And I'm so impatient. We had dinner and we go to this party and we go for a walk, and then I go home, and I'm thinking, "What's happening here?" He didn't make a move, and I was just dying of curiosity. So then I called him up the next day. And I said, "Was that a date?" [Laughs.] And so he loved that. He loved that—that I called and asked him that.

Then he explained that his long-distance girlfriend had just broken up with him, and that was not completely resolved. I did not feel compelled to explain all of my little involvements. So then we started dating, and then he kissed me.

INTERVIEWER: What was that like for you, when he kissed you?

As Hadley had previously stressed that she only felt sexually respon-
sive to women and couldn't imagine physical closeness with a man, the
interviewer picks up this incident and invites Hadley to reflect on her
emotional experience by asking what the kiss "was like" for her.

HADLEY: Oh, it was really sweet. He's a really sweet guy. And
I was very nervous about the kiss, right, like the kiss that I
was waiting for. I had already decided that I needed someone to make a move on me. Besides, I was worried that if
I made a move on a guy, I would say, "Yuk!" Anyway, he
walks up to me, kisses me, and I was so shocked, it was so
sudden.

INTERVIEWER: And you didn't go "Yuk?"

Here we see how closely the interviewer is in tune with Hadley, picking
up the words of her imagined fear. This intervention leads to a very long
narration, uninterrupted, in which Hadley details the emerging relation-
ship with Daniel and its course over the next 3 years.

Good Interview 3

The third interview comes from a study of the growth of self-
esteem. The interviewer, expecting "good moment" stories, was
quite unprepared to hear about traumatic experience. Being a highly
sensitive interviewer, she nicely circled around the trauma, gently
dealt with the painful emotion that arose, and ended up with a very
powerful and revealing interview.

The participant, Anneliese, was a woman in her mid-30s from
Holland. The interviewer was a somewhat younger Canadian
woman.

INTERVIEWER: I would like you to tell me about a period in
your life that made you feel better about yourself.

ANNELIESE: Yes. I think that when my father died, he had
lung cancer and was very sick, and that's it. I went there for
3 months.

This is a surprise to the interviewer, who is expecting a more upbeat sort of response. But she carries on to hear the story, keeping in mind the anchor of her question about self-esteem, and curious about how this story might relate to self-esteem.

INTERVIEWER: When was this?

Clarification to orient the story.

ANNELIESE: It was 2 years ago, and I was with him the whole time that he was sick—from the minute that we heard until he died. It was 3 months, it was very quick, but it was good for me. I saw that I could do something, that I could be with him. That's really one of the things that made a big change for me. It was special, because I had the feeling I could show him I was a good daughter. And it was also for myself, because I felt so sorry that he was sick and had nobody, it was difficult.

INTERVIEWER: So he was there by himself, and you came for 3 months by yourself?

Empathic question, summarizing the central factual aspects of the story so far.

ANNELIESE: With my daughter, but it was very difficult, because he was very sick and I could not speak to him. It was a very traumatic experience for me, because it was the first time in my life that I was confronted with somebody dying. It was also for me an experience that, in a way, that this is how things go. I grew up, and he died, and that's it, I'm left behind . . . life goes on. That's life. That somehow changed me. I became more mature, more serious in life.

INTERVIEWER: More serious?

Here the interviewer picks up, empathically, the piece of the story that relates to the issue of feeling good about the self. If the research topic were about grief or mortality, the interviewer would respond differently.

ANNELIESE: So this is definitely . . . also becoming a mother made a big difference in me. My father and my child, these are the most important things in my life that happened that changed me in a way, positively. Even though the death of my father was very, very hard. Not the time that I was there, because I was too busy running around. The hospital, the funeral, and this and that; you know, all sorts of obligations that you have in that time. But when I came back to Canada and I was confronted with my husband and I came back to my normal daily routine, suddenly I got the big fall and then I was very depressed, but you get over it.

INTERVIEWER: So even though it was a hard time for you, you still tell it as something that made you feel better about yourself.

The interviewer is empathically responding, and also linking and reorienting to the little q interview question.

ANNELIESE: Yes, yes, yes. I do. It is not a very nice experience, but anyway, it happens. In a way I realized the circle of life, and it was his time to go. But it was also good for me to show him that in his last days I was there for him. And this, I think, was the most important thing. I think he realized that, and this made us much more close.

INTERVIEWER: So you got close before he passed away?

Another empathic question.

ANNELIESE: Yes.

INTERVIEWER: So was that something that you did not have much of before that?

Now the interviewer is at a choice point. The main point of the previous narration has been "being there for him," but the interviewer pursues the story of the relationship to the father, perhaps trying to understand more about how getting close to her father is linked to feeling good about herself.

ANNELIESE: Not, not really. My parents were divorced when I was 6, and I grew up with my mother in Holland. I saw my father once a year, so we weren't close. Later in life, when my daughter was born, he came to Canada every year and visited us, but there were still some things that I couldn't really understand. When he died, I was looking through his things, and I found his diary. I saw a, that in a way he was also a person with a lot of emotions, but he was not . . . now I finally understood that he was not the type of person to open up. [She starts crying.]

INTERVIEWER: It's hard.

Empathically mirroring her emotion.

ANNELIESE: Yeah, well, it's okay. [Pause] So, anyway, I was going to throw his things away, and in a way I got to know him. [Crying]

INTERVIEWER: Maybe we can move to talking about your daughter, and then, when you feel comfortable, we can move back.

It is hard to know without being there if it is necessary to move away from what Anneliese is talking about at this point, but the interviewer trusts her own sensitivity and handles this deftly. It is commendable that she gives the participant a choice here.

ANNELIESE: My daughter is a change in my life that made me feel better about myself, because . . . in a way you're not alone any more, and it is also a responsibility, and any decision that you make, she is the major factor that you decide what to do and if to do, and it is also a person that is so close to you, so attached to you, that loves you if you are good or bad, without any interest in that. This is one of the most beautiful things in life.

INTERVIEWER: It sounds like you are talking about a few things. About responsibility and about an unconditional love.

This is an effort to be empathic, but the interviewer moves to a more intellectual level and away from Anneliese's strong emotion, which Anneliese marks in the ensuing "maybe."

ANNELIESE: Yes, maybe. I grew up with my mother and my sister. My sister was 10 years older than me, so I was the little one, and in a way I was always being kept. Well, until today, it's normal. But maybe that's why when I finally had a child of my own, I was like, "There, you see, you can finally take responsibility." There are other things in life, like opening my business or finishing my studies, that made me feel good, like "Yes, I can do it." It is many things, but, like I said before, the most dominant were the death of my father and the birth of my child.

INTERVIEWER: It is interesting you brought your child with you to your father in his last days, and you bring them both as . . .

This is a very interesting, but unnecessary, process comment, in which the interviewer is trying to call to Anneliese's attention the parallel of Anneliese's bringing her child and father into the interview. But she doesn't get to finish it, because Anneliese is quite engaged with her story, which she wants to continue to tell.

ANNELIESE: Mmm-hmm, yes, absolutely. I knew when I was going there that it could take 1 or 2 or maybe 6 months, so it is difficult to leave her behind, and second of all, I wanted her to see him. Her name, Terenia, is a Polish name, and I did it for my father, so this was important. She also learned the language and got to know my father's family, which is very important. Something like passing my identity to her.

INTERVIEWER: It seems identity is important to you—through your father, your daughter . . .

Empathic response.

ANNELIESE: Yes, absolutely. Because my mother had a difficult life. If you hear her story, it is amazing, you could make a movie of her, and we never had a feeling of having a home or having a family; that's why it was so important to me that my daughter would not have that. But of course my mother was from a different generation, different times. Of course, the Second World War, Holocaust, and all these things, and it is understandable. We are a different generation, new times. And for my identity, the period that he died was hard, but very positive, because for me that was a period that was over. Although it sounds strange, it was positive in a way, because when I came back I could not blame myself for anything. I went there, I was there for him, I did everything I could, I could not do better, and my sister until today has bad feelings of guilt that I don't have.

INTERVIEWER: Do you see anything that has changed in the way you feel about yourself since you came back from being with your father?

This is a clarification request. The interviewer is asking Anneliese to specify meanings in relation to the Big Q question about self-esteem.

ANNELIESE: Yes. I became more tough in a way, because I realized, as I told you before, that things happen to people, it is a very natural thing. When I came back home, it was, like, "Okay, now I am grown up."

INTERVIEWER: It sounds like being grown up is important to you.

The interviewer has now clarified to her own satisfaction that a key theme here is "being grown up," and she offers her understanding of this in an effort to get Anneliese to enlarge this theme.

ANNELIESE: Yes, and through the death of my father and the birth of my daughter, I know that. I mean, my mother, after the divorce from my father she was doing all she can, sometimes more than she can. But with my father it was different . . .

From here, the interviewee began what became a four-page narration in the transcript, detailing both her family history and the history of her relationship with her father. Anneliese was revealing her intense and conflicted emotions in this turbulent family history, but she did not lose emotional control. Note that the interviewer's capacity to contain the interviewee's emotions—neither pushing her nor running away—was what seemed to have made this very revealing narration possible.

Common Threads

What is common to these very different good interviews is that the interviewers have created a responsive and accepting relationship with their interviewees, whom they have brought into connection with their research question and then offered an experience-near starting point. They have adopted an empathic attitude and do an excellent job of staying with their interviewees. As I have tried to indicate in my commentary, there are choice points. There is not a single way to do it "right," and the choices are made in terms of what will further the inquiry and stay in contact with the narrator at the same time. Conducting and reviewing at least one pilot interview (see Exercise 6 below) will give you valuable practice in making such choices.

Exercise 6. Conducting and Reviewing a Pilot Interview

For those just beginning to conduct interviews, and for those beginning a new project, a supervised pilot interview (maybe even more than one) is very important. Find someone who fits the classification of those you want to study, and try out an interview with him or her. (You may need to get your IRB's permission to do this.) After you transcribe the recording, bring it either to your supervisor or to a collaboration group of peers and go over the interview minutely, looking at the dynamics of the interaction rather than the content of what you learned about the question. Look for places where you were smoothly in contact with the participant and moments where you shifted the topic, missed an important thread, or interrupted the flow. Try to reconstruct what may have been going on in you at such moments. If anxiety got you off balance, what was creating the anxiety? If you didn't know a better way to respond, think together about some alternatives that might have suited the moment.

CHAPTER 8

Learning from Bad and Difficult Interviews

*B*ad qualitative interviews are ones that devolve into question-and-answer format. Rather than being invited to offer their own constructions of their world (in relation to the research question), participants are being asked to respond to the interviewer's structures. Participants are being mined for answers rather than actively encouraged to tell the stories that are meaningful to them in their lives. Interviews can also go bad because a cooperative interchange has not been established in the relationship. The interviewer may be leading or judging, and on analysis, it will be hard to know whose meanings the narrative text reflects. This chapter presents some examples of interviewing mistakes, with commentary.

Simple Interviewing Mistakes

The following excerpts are from a study of adolescent development focused on the sense of time in relation to activities. The conceptual question concerned how free time both constructs and reflects identity. The little q question was designed to launch each teenage participant into a narrative about his or her activities and how they were meaningful. Both interviewer and interviewee in this case were male. The interviewer was inexperienced and quite anxious. In this example, we can see the interviewer making many of the mistakes common to novices.

Interrupting with Premature Requests for Clarification

> INTERVIEWER: Tell me about things that you like to do. Tell me something about yourself, about your friends.

> JOHN: Usually I come home from school and there isn't much . . .

> INTERVIEWER: When do you return from school?

Although the interviewer begins with an easily grasped little q question appropriate for teenagers, the interviewer's anxiety leads him to interrupt with another question before the interviewee has even gotten started. This request for clarification is premature and distracting.

Interjecting a Question Unrelated to the Narration

From a later point in the same interview:

> JOHN: I study for exams, and then there isn't much time to meet with friends, but now, you know, when there is less pressure, I meet my friends in the evening. We are going . . .

> INTERVIEWER: How old are you?

The interviewer interrupts John with an unrelated question.

Asking Yes-or-No Questions

> JOHN: I am among the older ones in my class, but that's okay. The difference in age doesn't bother me.

> INTERVIEWER: Do you feel that you have places to go?

Here we clearly see that the interviewer is turning this into a question-and-answer format. In addition, asking a yes-or-no question is unlikely to lead to rich detail.

Interrogating

Later, John talks about going out to parties and movies, but the interviewer responds with an interrogation:

> INTERVIEWER: Who is giving the parties? Who organizes them? Where do they take place?

The interviewer must never sound like a prosecutor firing questions.

Answering One's Own Question

> JOHN: Like last weekend, I was at this party, and it was so crowded . . .
>
> INTERVIEWER: So what do you do there? Dance and sit at the bar?

There is no justification for putting one's own imagination into the interview space, except in rare instances where one wants to invite the participant to correct one's own preconceptions. In this case, however, the interviewer seems unable to listen to what John wants to tell.

Asking Unanswerable, Experience-Distant Questions

> INTERVIEWER: How would you define yourself? Do you define yourself as being sociable? Do you have a lot of friends?

This is a string of unanswerable questions. I immediately wonder: What does it mean to "define yourself"?

Do people commonly "define" themselves, and if so, under what circumstances and to whom? What does it mean to "define yourself" as "sociable"? And how many friends is "a lot"? Interviewees might try to comply with such questions and try to answer them, but such questions are not likely to evoke meaningful material—or to create a collaborative relationship.

Focusing Responses on Facts Rather Than Meanings

JOHN: I am active in the Student Council.

INTERVIEWER: You mean at school?

JOHN: Yes.

INTERVIEWER: For a long time?

JOHN: This is the second year. In elementary school, I did a lot of clubs and things.

INTERVIEWER: But you moved to this school in grade 9, right?

JOHN: Yes.

INTERVIEWER: And from then on you are in Student Council?

JOHN: Yes.

INTERVIEWER: Are you elected to that?

JOHN: Yes.

How much more meaningful and inviting it would be simply to respond to "I am active in the Student Council" with "Tell me more about that" or "Tell me how you came to be doing that."

Expecting the Interviewee to Answer the Research Question

JOHN: I was active in the student volunteer program of the Red Cross. I had some free time—I guess I could have studied more, but I felt I could join something else and do some interesting things related to health care.

INTERVIEWER: Would you say that having free time is the reason you joined the Red Cross?

Here the interviewer/researcher is asking John to ratify some conceptual-level conclusion that he, the interviewer, is thinking about. He asks, in effect, whether free time was the cause of John's joining the Red Cross. Indeed, this narration is very close to the topic of interest in this research. In order to explore it, he would have to invite further narration through reflection: "So you had some free time and thought that joining the Red Cross would be an interesting way to use it."

Difficulty in Finding the Empathic Stance

The excerpt below is from a class exercise project that investigated the inner experience of maintaining a (doctoral) student role while working in a professional role. In this segment, we can see the interviewer's difficulty in finding an empathic stance. It is not so much that the interviewer was completely wrong in her understanding, but she was not tracking the development of the material in the interviewee and was inserting her own ideas. Although she might be obtaining a general idea of the dilemma that this interviewee experienced, she was missing thick description of experiences.

> INTERVIEWER: My question is, what is it like having two roles? For example, being a full-time student and then being full-time something else, like a full-time teacher. What is that experience like for you?
>
> *This is a good beginning, introducing the experience-near question and inviting the participant to reflect on her experience.*
>
> PAULA: It's much more challenging than I initially thought it would be, especially the full-time student role, because I really hadn't thought about it. I was only kind of framing it initially . . . as far as employment roles. I didn't think about all the other roles we have too. Initially, when I first started my doctoral program, I thought, "Gosh . . . I have all these resources. I've got the same time situation in that

I teach college, so I have my summers free." I thought it would be a piece of cake. I thought, "Wow . . . I can really wrap this up in 3 years." I know that it is very unusual, and now I'm at the end of year 6. So, you know, I just envisioned it going much more differently. I would manage this other role much more efficiently, and it's not that I think it's been inefficient, but it's a much more . . . it uses a lot more resources than I ever thought it would. I find that being in the role of a student . . . in itself is like a narcissistic injury. You know, you are in the role of not knowing and having to excavate that information with support and plenty of resources, but it's still very difficult and constantly being at the bottom of the learning curve. I feel like I'm constantly learning new things. I'm constantly being put in the role where I am not the expert. My weaknesses are being exposed. My lacks are being . . .

INTERVIEWER: You're vulnerable . . .

Here the interviewer interrupts the participant needlessly and introduces her own word ("vulnerable"), which is not part of Paula's narrative.

PAULA: Yeah, very vulnerable. So all of that is right there out on the surface, and that is very different from the roles I'm expected to take elsewhere. Like, professionally, I'm expected to be confident. I'm expected to be the one people go to. Especially . . . I mean not especially, but I can see that in the classroom I'm expected to know this body of knowledge and I do, but do I know everything about it? Of course not, because I'm also spending time in the classroom digging up more. I guess the reality is I'll never know all of it. I practice in the realms where I feel very proficient, and I build up my weaknesses, but still it is very hard to keep those things separate and to remain confident in those other roles when you realize there is still so much to know, and attention is constantly being drawn to how much you don't know, so I think it is difficult to try to maintain those two roles.

Notice that although Paula superficially agrees with the word "vulnerable," she doesn't really elaborate it and instead resumes her own direc-

tion. *Note that she elaborates the idea of "weakness" and talks about how she feels it seeping into her role as a teacher.*

INTERVIEWER: You said as a student you felt vulnerability. As a teacher, did you experience the same kind of vulnerability?

Now it is clear that the interviewer is following her own idea rather than the participant's and seems not to hear the deepening material around the experience of "not knowing," which Paula says pervades her role as a teacher as well. Note also that the interviewer asks a "closed," yes-or-no question rather than an invitation for further elaboration. In addition, Paula has already begun to discuss her experiences as a teacher, and it seems that the interviewer here is thinking about the vulnerability issue and not listening.

PAULA: Well, it's inevitable for some of that stuff to bleed over, if you are not very vigilant about it. So, just in my experience of myself maneuvering around that role, that I am aware that I don't have my PhD and I'm teaching at the university. I feel like everyone else does. Well, guess what? Not everyone else does. That's the reality of it, but my . . . in my imagination . . . my fantasy of it is that everyone knows more than I do . . . just like in my student role. So I really have to try to keep that fantasy in check and remember that not everyone knows more than I do, and that I do have a lot to offer and that I do know a lot about what I know . . .

Possibly in response to her sense of not having been listened to, Paula shifts to talking about herself in the second person ("you"), and then begins to question whether her experience is indeed universal. She does, however, then go back to trying to clarify her two experiences—one of knowing less than others, and the other of having a lot of knowledge.

INTERVIEWER: Because you're a teacher. You have an expertise.

Here the interviewer interjects perhaps some kind of admiration, but there is no call for admiration here—and she is again interrupting.

PAULA: Right. I have an area of expertise, and so I find myself

struggling at times with that . . . with the duality of that
. . . with being . . . having all these "lacks" and these weaknesses being exposed, and at other times having to act with
confidence, because you do have to act with confidence. I
mean, otherwise, you won't be able to effectively do your
job, and you will always second-guess yourself. So I guess
that my internal struggle is having a foot in both worlds.
Sometimes I'm the expert and sometimes the novice. So
that is difficult . . .

INTERVIEWER: It sounds like it hasn't gone as quickly or as
smoothly as you thought.

Following this very clear and perceptive narration that Paula
offered about herself, the interviewer inserted something unrelated
rather than asking for particular experiences that might illustrate
the general themes. This might be a good moment to get to more
detail by asking the participant how she decided to take up being
a student again and how that experience has evolved in relation to
her teaching role. Or the interviewer could ask for a story of a time
when Paula particularly experienced "having a foot in both worlds."

It is also important to notice here that, with some interviewees,
the interview will proceed despite the misdirection of the interviewer. Once the interviewee is fully in contact with the interviewer's question and calls up the story he or she wishes to tell, the
impetus is to tell it. But the interviewer can't count on this in all
instances. Although I certainly don't advocate poor interviewing
technique, it is not necessarily fatal to the interview or the material
that may be produced. (Of course, at the analysis stage, to speak in
terms of "vulnerability" in regard to this interviewee would then
become bad analysis.)

Fearing the Interviewee's Pain

When the interviewee gets close to painful feelings, the interviewer
has to be prepared to contain and be with whatever emotion arises.

Unless the interviewee is very traumatized or fragile, the feeling will be experienced and expressed, and then it will pass. But, out of fear, some interviewers feel a need to distract the participant from his or her own feelings or to offer some kind of pep talk. This kind of response always closes down the interview to full exploration and may be experienced as patronizing. The following excerpt comes from a study about the experience of immigration, so loss was very likely to be an important issue.

> PARTICIPANT: When I left home to come to the U.S., I realized that it was the end, that I'd never see my wonderful friends again, that our little group that had such fun together, it was over, done. It would never be the same [tears welling].
>
> INTERVIEWER: But now there is Skype and Facebook, so you can keep in touch.

Of course Skype and Facebook now exist, and the interviewee was likely well aware of this—but the interviewer here signaled that she didn't want to explore the pain of loss with the interviewee, even to understand better what was lost. An empathic response would be a kind, gentle "It would never be the same," thus reflecting the sadness, or "They became part of a lost world," which might extend an exploration of what was lost. Silence might also be appropriate—just sitting through the interviewee's flood of feeling until she was ready to resume her narration.

Letting One's Own Assumptions Get in the Way

An interview can get off track (or may never get on track) if the interviewee rejects the researcher's premises in a question. In another interview from the study of immigration mentioned above, the initial (little q) question was offered as "I'd like you to tell me about some of the difficulties you had when you first came to this country." The first response was "Well, I wouldn't say I had any difficulties. It all went very well." Notice that "difficulties" was not a word that, for reasons the interviewer could not yet understand, the participant used to understand his own experience. At this point, the interviewer needed to understand better the overall frame of how this participant thought about his immigration experience before locating the kinds of experience of interest to the research. The best response here to keep the interview moving forward would be "Okay. Then please tell me the story of your immigration. How did it come about, and what are the main things you remember about your early experiences in this country?" Perhaps the interviewee needed to have his successes mirrored before talking about his struggles, and the interviewer was now being signaled to move carefully here. In any case, the word "difficulties" would ideally not be used again in this interview; the researcher would need to be alert for what kind of language the interviewee used to note moments of challenge or struggle, and would need to make use of these.

We all make assumptions. This is not a problem if interviewers don't insist on them and are prepared to put them aside to join their participants' meanings.

Letting Previously Formed Images Get in the Way

Here I return to the interview presented in Chapter 5 (pp. 88–90), in which the interviewer neglected to get details of an "out of control" period in the participant's life—even though it was clearly important to the question of the study. In the review of this interview, this student was chagrined about not having asked about the "difficult period," which she realized was important to know about in order to understand how her participant made the transition into a lesbian identity. "Why didn't I follow that?" the interviewer later wondered. I asked her to think about what might have been going on in her mind, but she remained mystified. Later, while we were talking about some other aspect of the interview, I learned that the participant had once been her yoga teacher. They hadn't gotten to know one another, so my student thought it wasn't problematic to have her be a participant. But in exploring this, we came to understand that her prior view of this woman as a "teacher" (someone who had herself in control and was well organized) interfered with her capacity to relate to and recognize another side to this woman (one out of control and in great distress). This was, of course, an unconscious process, but the student was able to recognize it with supervision.

The Difficult Interview

Interviews can be difficult for many reasons. Sometimes people agree to be interviewed, but then are chagrined when they realize the level of self-disclosure that is invited. Some people are just not very self-reflective and balk at the idea of sharing themselves beyond recounting the simply factual. Other people have an agenda and refuse to stray from whatever their prepackaged point of view may be. In all such cases, the researcher must, as a matter of ethics, maintain a respectful attitude toward the participants, hear out whatever they wish to tell, and thank them for their time and participation. And the researcher then has to be resigned to the possibility that such interviews may not have been very useful.

Still, if a participant has come to an interview, he or she has a story to tell. The researcher has to keep trying gently but persistently during the interview to find a pathway into the participant's experience. This may mean listening through some fairly superficial stories while trust and the relationship build, in hopes of moving on to more personally significant experience. Sometimes the interviewee will "test" the interviewer to decide whether the interviewer is worthy of being entrusted with personal, meaningful experience. This was the case in what I consider to be the most difficult interview I have ever supervised, or ever even read. I present it to demonstrate how the interviewer stayed the course through quite direct and pointed challenges and ended up with a rich and detailed interview.

The Most Difficult Interview I Ever Supervised

The project concerned the child survivors of the Holocaust who immigrated to Israel, and their experiences of recounting their Holocaust experiences over the course of their lives. The participants were all in their 70s or 80s. The interviewer/researcher, Sharon Kangisser Cohen, was, at the time of the interview, a woman in her late 20s who was quite knowledgeable about the Holocaust. In arranging the interview meeting with Leah, Sharon had explained that she was interested in learning about survivors' experiences in telling about what had happened to them. She was aware that most of the people she was going to interview had already recounted their Holocaust experiences to Yad Vashem, the Holocaust oral history archive. She explained that she would be mainly focusing on their experiences of telling others about their Holocaust experiences, rather than the experiences themselves. Sharon had chosen to use a form of life history interviewing that asks a participant to begin by dividing his or her life into chapters, giving each chapter a title, and then telling about the most significant events in the chapter. Many interviewees find this structure a useful way of organizing a life story.[1]

> LEAH: What do you want to start with?
>
> SHARON: Do you think you could you divide your life into a few chapters and . . .
>
> LEAH: What does that mean? Divide your life into a few chapters?
>
> *Sharon is interrupted before she even sets out the whole first question and is put on alert that the interviewee is approaching this interview in a challenging stance, ready to fight about something.*

---

[1]Many studies have been done using this "chapters" approach, but I never found it very useful and gave it up. Different interviewers are able to work with different formats, which is in part what makes standardizing so difficult. What matters most is to have prompts that will lead interviewers to the material they wish to access.

SHARON: How do you see your life? Are there a few chapters that you can identify and describe, or do you see it as one continual . . .

Sharon tries to modify the question to make it more acceptable, but is again interrupted.

LEAH: I can't answer a question like that. I am a person like everyone else. Do you ask yourself to divide your life into a few chapters?

SHARON: No.

Here Sharon is taken aback by the hostility and can't think quickly enough to respond to the central communication of "I am a person like everyone else." At the same time, in allowing Leah to turn the tables and ask the questions, she is signaling her willingness to try to find a way to talk to one another.

LEAH: You should know I am against when people put the people who went through the Shoah into boxes. Every time it is discussed on television, I call in and I am angry. We are ordinary people like everyone else. I have integrated just like a Sabra. My mother tongue is Hebrew; I did not have any difficulties in my absorption. I have a problem that I didn't have a childhood and I don't have a family. I don't have any aunts or uncles or cousins. I don't have that. But what I created afterwards . . . but to divide into chapters, that is unacceptable to me. It is unacceptable to put people into boxes, and they do that to people who experienced the Shoah. With every war, they say that for those who have been through the Shoah, they find the war more difficult. That's nonsense. It's unacceptable to me. I am an ordinary person like everyone else. The only thing is that I don't have family. It hurts me, and it is getting even more painful. I have children, grandchildren, everything, and I have my husband's family in Jerusalem. But what we are missing is family.

SHARON: When were you born?

Sharon here chooses to try to anchor the interview in some basic factual material, perhaps in hopes that they can find a way of being comfortable talking to one another. Another choice here might be to empathically pick up Leah's sense of loss of family, since that is the primary theme, but I think it would be premature to do this. There isn't enough rapport to support talking about such painful material at this point. Yet another choice might be to reflect the "I am a person like everyone else" theme with a summarizing comment like this: "So you've led a life just like all other ordinary people, but with a different early history that has led other people to treat you in ways that have made you feel put in a box." At least this would indicate to Leah that Sharon is hearing what she has been telling. Under the difficult circumstances of Leah's prickliness, though, we have to keep in mind that we can see this more easily with hindsight.

LEAH: I was born on 29th May, 1936, in Czechoslovakia, to parents who were academics. Who held academic degrees. That's it. When the Germans invaded, I was 4 years old, and then they took all the children and put them into a ghetto, and slowly, slowly, they had Aktionen and my whole family perished in the first Aktion, uncles, aunts, cousins, etc. I was in the ghetto for 3 years. Have you read about the Shoah?

SHARON: Yes.

*One can almost read Leah's thought process: "Who am I talking to? You are just a kid. Do you have **any idea** what my experience may have been like? Do you even **know** the basic factual history?" The "Yes" is enough reassurance for her to go on. It does not need elaboration, which might sound defensive.*

LEAH: The end of the ghetto began in 1942, when they began the children's Aktionen. Then I was already 7 years old. Something like that. They hid us. They hid me with a family who were later awarded Righteous Gentiles. I was hidden by a family who had friends who my father had taught at the university. I was with them for a year. My parents remained in the ghetto, and they were then taken to concentration camps. My sister was in the underground, and when the Russians liberated them, she came for me and we fled. After we roamed through Europe, Byelorussia,

Poland, and Hungary, we arrived in Romania. The war ended there in 1945, and, if you know, they divided Europe into a German part, an English part, a Russian part, and an American part. And we were in the Russian part, and the plan was to get to Constantinople and from there to Israel. But the Russians said that all of the Jews in the Baltic States are considered Russians and therefore are not allowed to leave. Therefore, we fled again, and we reached the British side. The British put us into transit camps. The Brigade arrived, and we were taken to Italy. In Italy the soldiers of the Brigade took us to the Italian zone. Do you know that the Brigade was part of the British Army? We spent 4 years in Italy in an institution for children which the Brigade had established. If you are interested in children of the Shoah, you should read Aaron Maggid's book. I was there. My mother was a doctor in that institution. The older children got certificates to go to Israel in order to fight in the war of independence. In November 1948, we made aliya to Israel.

SHARON: Do you have memories from the period of the Shoah?

The interviewer is here perhaps trying to encourage Leah to narrate more from her own history, but Leah overreacts to its clumsiness.

LEAH: Of course, I have. I have memories.

SHARON: Could you tell me some of them?

I think this is still too risky an area for so early in the interview. It also seems to be an aside from what they have agreed to talk about, which are the experiences of telling about Holocaust experiences. Sharon is here clearly unsettled and off balance in the face of Leah's forceful challenging.

LEAH: What, for example? What do you want to know?

SHARON: Memories that are more dominant, that are with you all the time, or perhaps with time you have remembered certain things, more or less . . .

The interviewer seems to be looking for a way to talk about Holocaust experience that is personal rather than simply factual, as in the historical recounting that the participant has offered.

LEAH: I remember everything.

SHARON: Are there certain memories that . . .

LEAH: I don't remember the names of children. That I don't remember. Only those who live in Israel. We have started to meet other children where each one tells how he/she survived. How each one of them fled from the ghetto . . .

SHARON: Are there things you remember as happier moments or . . .

Sharon still is trying to invite a specific memory, perhaps as a starting point for a narrative of personal experience, but it isn't working. When a participant deflects a question repeatedly, it is better to switch direction and ask about something else.

LEAH: I don't understand what you mean.

SHARON: I simply want to hear some of your memories—from the ghetto, from your home . . .

This is good, in part because Sharon puts herself into the question. She makes plain what she is trying to learn about with this line of requests for memories.

LEAH: That's a very difficult question for me. Have you already interviewed people?

Leah is picking up on Sharon's increasing anxiety and wonders whether it is simply inexperience.

SHARON: Yes.

LEAH: What have they said?

SHARON: Everyone has his or her own story.

LEAH: I don't understand what you want.

I can't imagine an interviewer being made more anxious than this, but Sharon answers simply and honestly.

SHARON: To hear about your experiences . . .

LEAH: What type of experiences does a girl of 5, 6, or 7 have? That he knows that the Germans are coming and they say,

"To work," and he needs to go and find refuge. We were older children, we didn't have a childhood. We knew that we had to stay alive, whatever it took. We simply did not go through the childhood stage. We didn't have a childhood. We were big children. So essentially that is what is missing. I have told you that a stage of my life is missing, childhood.

Leah here goes to generalized experience, indicating that she is not going to talk about her own personal experiences under these conditions, although she says quite poignantly that her whole childhood is missing. She is also growing more impatient and hostile. She signals that, relationally, she can find no connection at all. Sharon cannot possibly ask at this point, "So what is it like to be missing a childhood?" A less determined (and sensitive) interviewer might have just looked for a way to end the interview at this point. But Sharon persists.

SHARON: Did you go to school?

*This is **the** crucial question that opens the interview. On the face of it, it doesn't seem to follow. But I think that Sharon is using her empathic intuition here—intuition based on subtle cues from the participant, who has indicated her valuing of academic pursuits and education, as well as her wish to be regarded as a normal person. Sharon perhaps remembers that Leah began the interview by locating herself as the daughter of parents who were academics. It is clear to her from Leah's way of speaking that Leah is educated, so she must have gone to school at some time. Sharon finds here a specific question that refers to personal experience and enters the life history on a track that the participant would like to discuss.*

LEAH: No. I only started to study at the age of 12 when I made aliya. Twelve years old—go to seventh grade, and I was fine, except for English, till this day if you ask me how I did it, I don't know. Only that every time I had to write in English . . . "How many years have you studied for?" and I would say, "Six," and they would say, "How could that be? Someone who has an academic degree, how can it be that you only studied for 6 years before that, or 10 years, including the degree?" In the end, I realized that I didn't need to actually say the truth, so I wrote that I had studied for 8 years. How did I manage to go to school and keep up? It's something . . . I simply read a lot. Perhaps the standard of education was . . . I was in a Zionist youth movement. When I made aliya, it was only with my mother. The only people from the whole family who survived from the ghetto were my mother and my sister. My mother was a doctor, so she got temporary work . . . and I couldn't stay with her, so I stayed in Tel Aviv with some of her friends who studied with her at university. My father had studied in Berlin in the '20s. After that, after 2 years, my mother had received permanent employment, and we lived together . . .

From here, the participant went on to tell her life story with rich detail and no longer challenged the interviewer (see Cohen, 2005, for a full report on this interview).

What is most important about this interview for our purposes here is that, despite the fairly incisive challenges, the interviewer stayed with the participant, answering the interviewee's piercing questions simply and trying to find a subject for comfortable conversation. This turned out to be the topic of education, which then led to other topics and eventually to the focus of the interview—the experiences of telling about her Shoah history. The interviewer never returned to the "chapters" structure, because she found another way to elicit the life history material that she needed for the study. What makes this interview stand out for me is that I have never encountered a participant who was quite so contentious at the beginning of an interview. And I admire the persistence and sensitivity of the interviewer in staying with her. It is an excellent example of what I have earlier described as "containment." If, with the benefit of hindsight, we reflect on the relational dynamics, we can see that this participant wanted to be sure that her interviewer was able to regard her as a normal person and an educated person before she was willing to explore with her the traumatic aspects of her past. This may be a good lesson for other encounters as well.

Difficult Interviewees

The "Press Release" Interviewee

There are some interviewees—particularly people in positions of some prominence—who seem ready to be interviewed but will only offer what seem like press releases, or official versions of some aspect of themselves. The only hope of getting past the press release to some other aspects of the self is to completely accept what is offered, while internally keeping in mind that there is more. The interviewer in such instances must avoid directly asking about problems or conflicts, but can try to empathize with feelings. Once, in interviewing a press release sort of person who was telling me about yet another honor he had received, I commented empathically, "That must have been a moment of great pride for you." The participant was momentarily stopped in his tracks; he hadn't thought about feeling proud of himself. He went on to say, "Well, I wished my father could have been there. He would never have believed I achieved so much," and continued from there to a much more nuanced and revealing life history.

The Garrulous Interviewee

Another kind of difficulty is presented by the garrulous interviewee—one who gets cranked up talking, is warmed by the interviewer's interest, and just keeps telling stories that seem to go increasingly farther afield from the topic of the interview, or to repeat the same theme and to be told primarily to entertain the interviewer ("Oh, yeah, let me tell you about another time we really had fun . . ."). The interviewer must, of course, laugh in the appropriate places and be entertained, but also must figure out how to get the interview back on the track of the research question. In such instances, it helps to track one's own thought process clearly and out loud, and to lead the interviewee back to the primary question of the research: "Let's see. I'm going to try to relate your story back to the question we started

with. From what I understand, the main theme is that you . . ."
This kind of response reframes the amorphous story into a structure
and helps the interviewee understand what the interviewer wants to
know about and why. It restates the purpose for being there, without
in any way suggesting that the interviewee is off the topic (which
would be shaming). Conducting the interview in this way represents a continued effort to bring the interviewee into contact with
the research question, in hopes that he or she will be able to create
or recall stories that fit this purpose.

Often the talkative interviewee is overtalking about something
other than him- or herself, and a request to return to personal experience will refocus the material. One garrulous woman I interviewed
for my study of identity responded, when I asked her to tell me about
her family, with "Well, I have seven brothers," and then launched
into a very detailed description of her first brother (complete with
descriptions of his wife and children, his wife's family, his occupational concerns, etc.). I had the sinking feeling as an interviewer that
if she was going to do the same for all seven brothers, I'd end up with
a lot of material to transcribe and nothing very useful to my study of
identity—despite my recognition of the importance of relationships
to identity. Although I was certainly interested in how she defined
herself in relation to her brothers, I only needed to know about how
they were important to her, not about their whole life spaces. After
she indeed began a similar report on her second brother, I stopped
her and said, "Before you go on, perhaps you can tell me about your
relationship with your first brother. What was the last interaction you
had with him, and what did it mean to you?" This served to refocus
her on herself in relation to her brothers, rather than on runaway
stories about them. I could also have picked up the main aspect of
her feeling about her first brother in her relationship to herself, but I
couldn't discern from her story about him what this was.

The Distressed Interviewee

Sometimes an interviewee is in the midst of some personal crisis that dominates his or her thoughts and makes it impossible to

focus on the topic of the interview. Every avenue that the interviewer tries to pursue with this participant leads back to the recent life event, which is raw and overwhelming. In such instances, the interviewer must be kind and sympathetic, but must try to bring the interview to an end. The interviewer may make gentle efforts to see whether the interviewee can turn his or her attention to the topic of interest, but if the participant cannot do so at this time, the interviewer simply has to give up—diplomatically. This happens rarely, but it does happen, and sometimes one can still glean a bit of useful material anyway.

The Hostile Interviewee

What if the interviewee gets angry or challenging (as in the difficult interview with Leah, presented above)? The first task is to try to understand the basis of the hostility and address it directly. The interviewer should answer any challenging questions straightforwardly and nondefensively. Often the hostility or challenge is a response to what the interviewee thinks the researcher's underlying motives may be in interviewing people in his or her particular group: "You're just trying to show that all people with [e.g., bipolar disorder] are unfit for society—to write about how many problems we have and how we disrupt society."

Here is a possible response to a challenge like this: "Actually the opposite. What I'm trying to do is to document and understand the actual experiences of people with [bipolar disorder], in order to give a fuller picture to a society that often misunderstands people like this. Your agreement to talk to me is in the service of creating that greater understanding." This restates the contract (including the possible benefit to the participant), and firmly aligns the researcher on the side of understanding, rather than perpetuation of prejudice. If this doesn't seem to dispel the challenge, the interviewer might ask the participant, "Have I said something that gave you that impression?" and try to address directly some miscommunication that may have occurred.

In the difficult interview with Leah, above, Leah said fairly directly that she was angry about Holocaust survivors' being "put in boxes." The interviewer might have empathized with this and said,

> "Yes, I know what you mean by Holocaust survivors' being treated as different by society, and that is a part of what I'm trying to understand—to understand how this has affected you and the circumstances in which you have chosen to tell or not to tell about your Holocaust experiences. And I want to understand also the ways in which you are just like everyone else and not in any kind of box."

The relational implicit message here would have been that the researcher was on the side of understanding, and *not* on the side of the forces that create and perpetuate misconception and prejudice, while acknowledging that such forces do indeed exist.

The "Boring" Interviewee

Sometimes anxious participants try to stick with superficial, ordinary accounts, as though their message is "There's nothing at all special about me." The following is an example from a study of students who were the first generation in their family to go to college:

INTERVIEWER: Could you please tell me about your family?

PARTICIPANT: It is just a normal family.

INTERVIEWER: And who is in your family?

PARTICIPANT: Mother, father, sister. Just a normal family.

INTERVIEWER: Could you try to think back to your very first memory of your mother? Try to go as far back as you can until you find a specific memory.

PARTICIPANT: I can't remember anything from my childhood, before about age 10.

INTERVIEWER: That's okay. Just go back as far as you can. Age 10 would be fine.

The interviewer can then stay with the "earliest memories" prompt for each of the other family members, or see whether the earliest memory of the mother leads to other memories that involve the other family members enough to get a sense of the participant's family experience.

It is important to remember that everyone has a story to tell, but some people are afraid that no one will find it of interest. Your job is to stay attuned to the person and to invite specific stories long enough to allow the interviewee to be a person of interest to you.

CHAPTER 9

Dos and Don'ts
of Interviewing

*I*n this chapter I offer brief pointers. Some of them I have commented on before, but in my view they bear repeating; others
have been implied or touched on earlier, but are highlighted
differently here; and still others are new tips.

Do ask about the interviewee's experience, rather than for generalized sociological opinions.

To ascertain how a woman approaches mothering in terms of val-
ues, ask, "What about your child do you value most? What do you
think makes him [or her] a 'good child' in your eyes?" rather than
"How would you define a good child?" Sometimes it makes sense
to start with the general and then move to the interviewee's experience, but too often in qualitative research, interviewers do not move
past generalizations about experience. When an interviewee offers
a generalization, always inquire about how this is experienced in a
personal way.

☯ *Don't expect consistency.*

If you are doing a qualitative study, you already recognize that people have multiple planes of experience, and you are likely to be interested in making sense of this complexity. You may know intellectually that people have multiple voices[1] and may give self-contradictory accounts of their experiences, but you may still be surprised when you actually hear it. It is very bad form in interviewing to say to an interviewee in an accusatory way, "You are contradicting yourself!" You may want to investigate issues of inconsistency by asking about what seem to you to be contradictions, but not in a way that suggests that there *ought* to be consistency. You can ask about how the seemingly inconsistent elements might go together in the participant's mind: "You've told me a number of times that you didn't feel much about losing your father at such a young age, and at other times, you've mentioned strong feelings of loss and anger. Can you help me understand how both of these are true for you?" This is a request for understanding what integration there might be of emotionally disparate states. In this example, the participant might explain that he or she has these experiences at different times or under different circumstances. Sometimes a participant cannot relate different experiences to one another, and this too is useful material for you, depending on your research question. Remember that the complexity is what you are pursuing. If you wanted simple and straightforward answers, you would just use a questionnaire.

☯ *Do inquire about linkages.*

Sometimes it may seem that a participant is "changing the subject," talking about one thing and then switching to a story about something else. Given that the mind associates what goes together, your

---

[1]Issues of coherence are complex theoretically. See especially Bakhtin (1981, 1986) and Linde (1993).

task at such times is to understand the connection. You might ask, when the second topic runs its course, "Can you tell me about how these things are linked for you? You were talking about *X* and then began telling me about *Y*, and I am wondering how you connected these things in your mind."

☯ Do track carefully and ask about what you don't understand.

Sometimes novice interviewers shy away from letting interviewees know that they don't understand some part of what is being told to them. This is always a mistake. Ask about what you can't follow. You can say something like this: "I'm afraid I'm a bit confused here, and I want to go over this again to try to understand better." It is important to own responsibility for not following, rather than to imply in any way that the interviewee is telling the story in a confusing way. (If you get a response like "I'm sorry, I wasn't clear," you are somehow subtly implying that it is the interviewee who is not meeting your expectations.) Many interviewees who get caught up in a memory, especially of a time that is marked by strong mixed feelings, jump ahead in their own minds and omit important details that would make their story make sense. Consider this example from a study of work–family balance in men:

> PHIL: The schools closed because of a snow emergency, and I knew I wouldn't get to work on time, if at all. My wife had a meeting that day she couldn't miss. Even if my coworkers were fine with my not coming in, which they typically were, I felt bad, because I felt like I was letting people down, and I don't do that well. So the choice was to be here with my kids and be resentful, to a certain extent, that I had to be here with them, which wasn't their fault. You know, it wasn't their fault they were 7 and 6 and needed adult supervision. So I called around to find someone to be with them, but couldn't find anyone. I knew that there

was important stuff happening that day. So then I went to the office.

INTERVIEWER: I'm confused here. So you went to your office leaving your kids at home alone?

PAUL: No, I took them with me for a few hours. But they were bored after a short time, and I didn't get much done.

It is probably Paul's anguish over this choice that leads him to tell this story with such a non sequitur ending, and it is important for the interviewer to say she is confused and to clarify what is confusing.

Do pay special attention to imagery.

If a participant offers an image or a metaphor in the narration, pay special attention to it by repeating it in an inquiring tone or asking for more thoughts about it. Images and metaphors contain revealing experiences that are not easily rendered in linear speech. For instance, here is a woman from my identity study talking about a period of transition:

LYDIA: It was a time of emerging. I felt like a butterfly.

INTERVIEWER (ME): Tell me more about the butterfly.

LYDIA: It was joyous. I felt like I had wings and could fly. I was breaking out of a cocoon. I had been living in Hawaii, and everything seemed possible. You know . . . before, I was doing all the things I was expected to do, but now I could pick where I would go. There were so many gardens to explore . . .

Don't ask hypothetical questions.

Questions like "How do you think you would have felt if such and such had happened?" do not produce useful material. The purpose of a qualitative interview is to learn about what *did* happen or what *was* felt or experienced or hoped for.

For example, this segment is part of an interview in a class exercise about people's relationships to animals. The interviewer has asked about pets, but the interviewee does not have a pet. Note what happens when the interviewer tries to pursue a hypothetical question.

> INTERVIEWER: If you would have a pet, if your life was organized in a way that a pet would fit in, what sort of pet would you choose to have?
>
> PARTICIPANT: Well, I don't think I would have a pet . . . but if pressed, uh . . . I'd rather just babysit other people's pets . . . I don't really think I want a pet. I'd take care of a dog . . .
>
> INTERVIEWER: A dog . . .
>
> PARTICIPANT: . . . But then . . . even as I'm saying that . . . I'm thinking, "What would I do for a week?" . . . I gotta be some place or gotta go some place.

We can see that the interviewee here resists getting hypothetical and goes back to his own experience. He also indicates that he feels "pressed" by the interviewer, which is not a desirable aspect of a research relationship. Indeed, hypothetical questions have the underlying structure of "If you were other than you are, then what . . . ?"

☯ *Don't make judgments.*

You are perhaps wondering why I repeatedly stress something as obvious as not making judgments, because of course you would never overtly criticize an interviewee. But positive comments like "That's great!" or "That's wonderful!" are also judgments, and I see them in my students' transcripts again and again. If you are making these kinds of evaluative positive comments, your interviewees become sensitive (even unconsciously) to *not* getting such responses to other aspects of their lives. Being nonjudgmental means not making judgments—either good or bad judgments. If you truly admire something an interviewee did or are truly happy for him or her, it is better to lodge such an emotional reaction, if appropriate, as an empathic response: "This sounds like something you were very proud of," or "So this gave you great pleasure." Affective joy expressed empathically with such responses is quite appropriate. In other words, you as the interviewer can overtly *feel* the positive feeling *with* the participant and smile or look joyous with him or her. It is not either appropriate or useful to express to a participant that something he or she felt was ordinary was "wonderful" in your eyes.

> PARTICIPANT: Last year I got the award as Nurse of the Year, but it was a political gesture and made all my colleagues suspicious of me.
>
> INTERVIEWER: Nurse of the Year Award!!! Well, I think that's wonderful. Congratulations!!!!

A better response might be this: "You got a major award, but it brought you trouble as well as pleasure."

☯ Don't take notes during the interview.

All the talk should be on the recording, so there should be no need for you to write. You will learn to pay close enough attention to what the interviewee is telling you to remember names of important people and places. If you forget, you can ask to be reminded. Note taking disrupts the relationship and calls attention to your different roles as the researcher and the participant, objectifying the participant. The participant wonders what you are writing and feels the shift in your attention. If there is something you feel you must write down lest you forget it, do so during a bathroom break, out of sight of the participant. One exception to this general rule is that if factual material or chronology is very important to keep track of, you might just keep notes of this as you are talking, making clear that this is what you are doing.

⊙ *Do invite the participant to ask questions or express concerns before you begin. Be transparent.*

It is better to respond to concerns about what will take place before the interview begins, so that the conversation can center on the topic at hand. It is unwise to suppress the participant's worry or curiosity. Often the questions posed at the beginning can have meanings that will sensitize you to areas that are vital for the participant.

One of the women in my longitudinal study asked me, at the interview when she was 58, how many of the original 30 women in my sample were still alive. It was no surprise, then, that I found that issues of mortality were very much on her mind.

Different interviewees require different degrees of transparency from you as they try to form an image of the person they are talking to. There is seldom a good reason to withhold information about yourself if it is requested. In my own experience, I am most often asked whether I have children or where I live, and I straightforwardly answer these questions.

It is fine to respond to personal questions, even if they may be about your personal connection to the group you are studying. Sometimes people will ask whether you know someone they know. If you do, it may make the participants feel more linked to you, but it may also raise particular confidentiality concerns, which you may then have to reemphasize. I think that no purpose is served by hiding behind some kind of professional mask here, although it is wise to try to be rather general in responding to personal questions if that will satisfy an interviewee.

⊙ *Don't know. Be unenlightened.*

Of course you want to present yourself as intelligent and competent. But people have their own meanings about things, especially aspects of the world in which they live. Resist the temptation to say that you already know about something they mention. Err on the side of asking for explanations. You can always say, "I've heard something about [e.g., the Rotary Club], but it would help me understand if you would explain to me its significance to you."

This extends to making assumptions about what words mean. People use words in different ways. If the participant is using a word repeatedly or placing emphasis on it, make sure you know what the participant means by it. Simply requesting is all that is necessary: "Tell me more about what you mean when you say your brother is 'weird.'" This holds true especially when participants try to use what they think is your language, perhaps psychological words. Their meanings are unlikely to be the same as your own. In the following example, it is a good thing that the interviewer does not take the participant's description at face value:

PARTICIPANT: My husband is bipolar.

INTERVIEWER: He was diagnosed with bipolar disorder?

PARTICIPANT: No, but, you know, his mood changes a lot.

🌑 *Don't cut people off or indicate that they are digressing.*

As I have stressed throughout this book, you have to hold on to both your interest in your research question and your interest in the interviewee, as well as to the link between these. You want your interviewees to tell their stories freely and in the form that makes most sense to them; at the same time, you want them to talk about matters related to what you are studying.

Especially if you are interviewing people who are isolated, people do sometimes take the opportunity to talk to an interested listener about whatever is on their minds. To advance the research relationship most effectively, you have to be primarily interested in the person and find ways to deftly steer the conversation back to the topic you have agreed to investigate together. Being impatient with digression will usually hurt people's feelings or shut them down altogether. Instead, try to find a smooth path from a digression back to the matters that you are interested in. You can do this by linking the digression back to what came before:

I understand that your daughter's upcoming wedding has claimed all your attention these days and kind of taken you away from the issues at school. You were telling me just before about how you felt about the new policies in your school and the impact they have on your decision about whether or not to continue to teach there, and I'd like to hear more about that.

Sometimes you may be trying to interview a participant who has a preoccupation, and every time you get close to that topic, the participant gets launched on a long story that is not useful for the research purposes. For example, one of the participants in my longitudinal study of identity formation had a long history of bosses she could not get along with, and she was still enraged at each one of them. She wanted to tell me in great detail about all of her grievances, and I had already understood well her sense of being misunderstood, misjudged, and mistreated. She had narrated three very lengthy, well-detailed accounts, so I had this material if I wanted to make use of such stories in their fine points. By the time she launched into her fourth such story, I commented that I understood that she had this experience quite a few times, and that I understood that this was very frustrating and painful for her. Then I said that perhaps we could now move to another area of her life, perhaps one in which she felt some success or satisfaction. Fortunately, after that, she was able to refer to these difficult work situations without getting immersed in them again—perhaps because she felt that I indicated that I understood how it was for her.

Don't ask questions out of curiosity unrelated to the research question you have defined.

Sometimes participants mention something that is of general interest to you but unrelated to the question you have agreed to talk about. A participant's agreement to talk to you about the topic (unless you have agreed to talk about a whole life history) does not give you license to ask them any question that comes to your mind just because you feel "curious." In other words, maximal curiosity about a participant's experience *in relation to your research question* is highly desirable in qualitative research; idle curiosity is impertinent. Here is an example from a study of parents of medically challenged infants:

> PARTICIPANT: We had excellent doctors who paid close attention to our son's problems. I think that my father being famous in this town helped get us the best possible doctors. But still we had to deal with the nightly care every 2 hours, never getting enough sleep ourselves, and the constant anxiety about whether he'd still be alive the next morning.

> *It suddenly dawns on the interviewer that his participant is the daughter of a well-known former football player.*

> INTERVIEWER: Oh—is your father _____? I used to watch him play. He was amazing. What was it like to grow up as his daughter?

This was out of bounds and likely to derail the interview, which was not focused on the participant's experiences of growing up in her particular family circumstances. And notice how unempathic the response was to the participant's talking about the challenges of an ill baby, which was, after all, the topic of the research. The interviewer allowed himself to become distracted from his own purposes. Under some circumstances, such unrelated questions can be unethical—taking advantage of an empathic research alliance in an exploitative way.

Do listen to yourself as an interviewer.

Often interviewers are not aware of being intrusive until they listen to their recordings. If you hear yourself talking over a participant, interrupting, or completing his or her sentences, stop and try to figure out why you were doing this. What anxiety were you experiencing that had you fighting to control the interview, rather than moving along with your participant? These may be moments to take for supervision.

☯ *Do welcome being corrected.*

If you use a word in a question or an empathic response, and the participant says, "Well, I wouldn't say it was _____," this is a good thing! Be grateful rather than defensive (although you can say, "Sorry if I misunderstood"). This becomes a platform for you to invite participants to detail the nuances of *their* meaning, to explain to you how you got it wrong, and to help you get it right.

> INTERVIEWER: So you're kind of coasting right now.
>
> PARTICIPANT: I wouldn't say it's coasting. I would say I'm trying to just calm down, waiting for that zest to kick in, waiting for that purpose to show up.

Here the participant corrects that her sense of calm waiting is different from coasting—that she is holding still rather than in motion.

☯ *Do be alert to negations, and investigate these.*

Sometimes interviewees will describe their experiences in terms of what they didn't feel or didn't think. It is important at such times to try to transcend these negations and ask for a description of what the interviewees *did* feel or think. Your empathic antennae must guide you here. You cannot empathize with absence of experience. Stay with it until you can feel it with a participant.

> PARTICIPANT: When my brother died, I didn't feel guilty. I wasn't sad. I didn't think much about him. I just went to the funeral.
>
> INTERVIEWER: You just went to the funeral. What were you aware of experiencing there?

PARTICIPANT: Just the futility of it all. It was a freak accident—could have happened to anyone or no one. Why was it him? Why not me?

The interviewer's attention to the negation and effort to elicit the experience rather than the absence of experience leads to illuminating material.

Do recognize that a lot of what is important cannot be put into words.

Annie Rogers and her students (Rogers, 2007; Rogers et al., 1999) have detailed a "language of the unsayable." Decoding this language means paying attention to negations, revisions, and smokescreens that mask feelings and experiences that cannot be put into words. Although these processes can sometimes be read at the analysis stage, you can often sense them as breaks in the research relationship as the interview unfolds. These are most likely to occur in relation to traumatized states. You may sense that it is not so much that the interviewee withdraws from talking to you as that he or she simply cannot access the experience. You may find that your attention is being redirected, or that you are becoming confused by unrelated details that are hard to organize. If this happens, you should try to clarify what you can, but at the same time must humbly accept that not all experience is narratable.

Don't offer commentary on the participant's life—even if invited to.

Your aim is to ascertain the participant's meanings, not to express your own. Sometimes, in talking about others in their lives, participants will ask for your opinion about these others—for example, "Don't you think that was a terrible thing for my sister to do?" You can respond with a facial expression or a head shake that matches the feeling, and simply repeat in the same tone of voice used by the participant, "Terrible." Or you can say, "It was terrible for you." Generally, what is being requested is acknowledgment rather than your assessment of the situation. Your job as the interviewer is to reflect the feeling.

In some instances, a participant may ask your professional opinion about someone else's behavior or possible mental health problems. The best response is that you just don't know and you wonder how *the participant* understands it. If you are pressed at the end of an interview, you can suggest resources for consultation if this seems necessary.

Sometimes an interviewee asks for (or looks for) some kind of feedback from you at the end of the interview: "I suppose you think I'm really strange, being this age and still [not being married, not having a career direction, having been in jail twice, having an addiction"—whatever it is]. It is important to be ready to normalize the experiences, whatever the participant has told you. You must say clearly something to the effect that many people are in the same boat, that you have heard about similar experiences from a number of others, that your own experiences are not all that different— whatever is honest and can encompass whatever the participant has told you as within the range of the human and understandable.

● *Do anticipate feeling unsettled at the end of the interview.*

In doing narrative interviews, you will always have more material than you think you have, as will become clear when you transcribe your recordings. If you are new to interviewing, you will leave your early interviews feeling that the participants have not fully "answered" your research question. That is to be expected. You, as the researcher, will be the one analyzing the data and exploring the research question, making use of the rich stories of experience you have obtained. You will also have other interviews to do to learn more. So don't mistake the postinterview letdown and confusion for some kind of failure. And don't prolong an interview in an effort to get everything settled.

If you are interviewing a person in distress, you may find your-self shaken by the interview. Many qualitative researchers report crying on the way home from an interview, because they are filled with another person's suffering (Granek, 2011; Gilbert, 2001). You can hope that your research may contribute to alleviating this suf-fering—not perhaps for your participant, but for others in the long run.

Do ask participants about their experience of their interviews.

Asking participants how they have experienced their interviews is an effort to continue, in Michelle Fine's (1994) phrase, to "work the hyphen" of the self–other divide by talking about how we are interrelated to and with our participants. Simply asking, "How has talking to me like this been for you?" is a way of reflecting together on the dynamics of the research relationship and may yield impor-tant material.

Do express your gratitude and say goodbye.

By the end of the interview, there may be a sense of an intimate bond between you, but you do have to say goodbye. This is espe-cially difficult with a participant who is isolated or lonely, but you cannot promise a continuing relationship. Here you can reiterate your role as a researcher, but indicate that the interaction has been meaningful to you and that you will continue to think about the participant. You may offer to send a copy of the results of your study if the participant wishes to have it. You may ask for permission to call if there turn out to be things on the recording that puzzle you. You offer your good wishes. The sadness of parting will pass for both of you. It is important to tell the participant how much you have appreciated his or her openness and honesty, and how much you have learned from him or her.

🌓 *Do practice.*

Work with a group of others who are learning interviewing skills, and do some role plays. Give and receive feedback. Pay attention to how present you (and others) are in engaging with your participants. Talk about moments of being out of contact, and discuss what created them. I cannot stress enough how important practice is. Interviewing is not a skill that people are born with; you have to give yourself opportunities to learn. You can also practice empathic responding while talking to your friends; they will begin to think of you as a great listener!

🌓 *Do report the context and nature of the interview when you write about your findings. Both what and how you ask shape the material.*

All too often, after carefully attending to the interview dynamics, researchers simply report their findings from interviews as though the material was somehow just there and they retrieved it. If you want to quote parts of the interview in your discussion, it is also important to include what interventions or prompts of yours the interviewee is responding to.

I participated in a group in which five qualitative researchers analyzed the same interview, each from our own methodological vantage point (Wertz et al., 2011). One point that provoked a great deal of discussion in our group turned on this very issue. The interview we were considering was carried out by an inexperienced peer of the interviewee, "Teresa," who was a psychology student who had been a rising opera singer until she lost her voice to thyroid cancer at the age of 19. She had been describing, quite eloquently, her experiences of loss. The transcript below picks up in the middle of the interview:

> TERESA: . . . That was difficult . . . healing physically and coming to terms with the fact that things would have to be

so different from then on . . . I wasn't even myself any more after that. My voice was gone, so I was gone, and I'd never been anything but my voice. So yeah, that was really hard.

INTERVIEWER: Since you did a lot of singing with yours and other churches, how did this affect your relationship with God?

*It is important to note that Teresa has not mentioned God at all to this point. This is the interviewer's assumption that she even **has** a relationship with God, and, as you will see, this confuses her.*

TERESA: That's an interesting question.

This response seems to signal that Teresa has to orient herself to the question. It does not resonate with her experience and is not a question to which she can readily respond.

INTERVIEWER: I mean, you worked for the church, and you were no longer able to . . .

TERESA: Yeah. That's a very interesting question. Well, for as long as I can remember, I've been a Catholic cantor, so I knew the Mass parts backwards and forwards, and I always had to stand at the front and lead the congregation, and everybody looked at me and thought, "Oh, isn't she a good Catholic," bla bla bla, and that's great. To be honest, if I wasn't singing, I wouldn't have gone to church. My relationship with God back then was . . . um . . . a casual, conversational one. I mean, it was, "Hi, God, how are you . . . I'm fine . . . that's good . . . how've you been . . ." and it suited me. And I was grateful for things, and I'd offer prayers of thanks. And then when this happened, and I couldn't sing . . . Obviously, I was initially grateful . . . grateful to be alive, grateful we'd caught it. Still freaked out, though, because the doctors kept telling me they hadn't gotten it all, that I had to be irradiated and have things burned out, and so forth. . . . The funny thing is that none of the churches I sang at were actually *my church*. They were paid jobs . . . I sang at a Catholic church, a Jewish temple, an Episcopal church, and a Baptist church.

I tried to go to church after surgery, just to go, but would have to leave during the opening hymn because I couldn't handle it. And then I started asking questions . . . not so much questioning God . . . but questioning religion in general. I got into studying East Asian philosophies, I got into studying all kinds of religious systems and beliefs . . . and I came to the conclusion that my relationship with God, as far as I'd always known it, was very much centered on my voice and being able to sing. And it was very real to me. Singing was my prayer. That was my connection. That was my big gift. I was a fat kid with no friends for as long as I could remember . . . but I could sing! That was the "in" for me. When I lost that, I lost my connection with God, I lost all my friends, I lost my calling in life, I lost my passion in life, I lost my trump card . . . the thing that was gonna get me out of being that fat kid with the oppressive dad, and whatever . . . that was going to be my ticket out. I lost my ticket! So I lost my connection to God. Gone. I began to understand things in a very logical, philosophical way, and I took to logic because passion hurt too much. Because music was passion for me. If I had a problem in life . . . seriously . . . I would sing. That's how I fixed it. Always. And I've had problems. Um . . . because I'm lucky like that. But I couldn't sing, even though things would happen. Like, uh, if I was dating a guy . . . and it wasn't like I would just date a guy. I would date a guy who'd beat me up. I was good like that. If I could sing, that would go away for me. Yeah. Couldn't sing. That was bad. Eventually, as my voice started trying to come back, I realized . . . I wasn't angry at God . . . I just really didn't think there was a god working on things for me out there. I don't have any animosity towards religion, nor do I have any judgments on people who have religious beliefs . . . I respect spirituality, I believe myself to be spiritual . . . yet I can't say that I now adhere to any one given faith. Qualifiedly agnostic, you could say. I'm open . . . if the deity of choice wants to zap me and give me a moment of epiphany, I'm fine with that. But as of yet, it hasn't occurred, to my knowledge. I'm waiting for whatever. In the meantime, I'll keep reading my Lao Tsu, and my Bhagavad Gita, and my Koran, and my Book of Mormon . . . I've got an interesting collection at home. But I keep myself abreast of the thoughts out there, and I think about it a lot . . . I do feel that spirituality is a big part of what I do, like in my writing, my music now . . . yeah. A huge part of it. I'd rather think of how I live and how much I live, though, rather than whether or not a greater being. Is there a god I'm giving it all up to? No, I don't feel that way. I feel that, honestly, if there's a god, and I end up in heaven, the first thing I'd like to hear is "Okay, you were wrong . . . I exist. But it's okay." I think that, if there is a god, he'll totally understand where I'm coming from . . . I think he'd be okay with it.

Teresa worked very hard to put her spiritual beliefs in terms she thought her interviewer, who seemed evidently to have another idea about God, could understand. If we read this excerpt carefully, we see that Teresa was in dialogue with the interviewer's assumption that his conception of God was the same as her own, and she was working to disabuse him of this idea. At the point of analysis, we must understand her narration in this context. In other words, she was explaining her relationship to God in some kind of opposition to what she thought her interviewer was taking for granted. We can strongly suspect that her narration would have been quite different if the interviewer had asked her how her loss affected her spiritual beliefs or her sense of her place in the universe. Teresa might then not have spoken about God at all.

Gary Gregg (2006), in his study of deep structures of identity, uses his reflections on the interview in a useful way: ". . . the interview has a jumpy quality that renders Mr. Bororo's views unnervingly incomplete and inconsistent. The researcher's questions cause some of this, but Mr. Bororo also shifts continually among the groups he contrasts as heavier- and lighter-drinking, and thus among the qualities he imputes to his group of traveling trouble-shooters" (pp. 65–66). Note here how Gregg uses his evaluation of the structure of the interview as part of his analysis and also assigns appropriate responsibility to the interviewer, at least letting his readers know that he has paid attention to what part of the interview material may have been a function of the interviewer. Reports on interview data must consider the relational context in which the material was obtained.

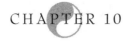

CHAPTER 10

After the Interview

*T*he first task after the interview is to record all of your impressions that were not part of the dialogue recorded. These include observations of the interviewee, your own feelings and reactions, and any thoughts or insights that may have occurred in relation to the question. If you met in your interviewee's home, make notes about the setting. Jot down something to remind you of what the interviewee looked like. You may also note comments the interviewee made before the recording began or after it ended, because these are often highly significant. You can either speak all these impressions into your recorder or write them down. Do not let time pass before doing this, because these observations are fleeting and vanish from memory quite quickly.

Transcription and Analysis

The best process for doing narrative research is to regard interviewing, analyzing, and conceptualizing as part of a circle that you orbit in each instance (Ouellette, 2003). The interview may provoke new thoughts about your research question and lead you back to the scholarly literature to see whether others have commented on what you have noticed or learned from your interview. A preliminary analysis of the interview you have just conducted will make the next one better.

I recommend transcribing the interview just after it was conducted. This makes it easier to review the interview and conduct an initial thematic analysis—or at least to reflect on what you have learned from the interview. I like to do my own transcription, as this puts me back in the interview moment, when I can pause and reflect on what I am hearing in a way that I couldn't do with the participant in front of me. But transcription is time-consuming, and you may prefer to hire someone else (who has signed appropriate confidentiality agreements) to do it. In such cases, you might listen to the recording along with the transcription—in part to check the transcription for accuracy, and in part to hear once again the participant's voice (as well as your own voice).

It will certainly be important to transcribe verbatim all the words on the recording, as well as sounds that indicate feelings (laughs, guffaws, sobs). These include speech markers ("um," "I don't know," etc.) that may reflect uncertainty or anxiety. You can also notate the tone of voice (e.g., "She sounds happy," "His voice is sad," "She speaks hesitantly"). Long pauses should also be indicated. Beyond this, the exactitude of transcription depends on what you intend to do with the data. I tell my students that if they don't intend to analyze the exact length of pauses, there is no need to time them. Many researchers who do discourse analysis have created complex and exacting transcription conventions, which may be used for analyzing the language and speech patterns of the interview (Willig, 2003; Potter & Wetherell, 1987). For other purposes that focus on meanings, you will have to transcribe with the aim of capturing the words used and meanings intended by the speaker. The hesitancies and uncertainties in speech that you may have noticed in the transcriptions in this book are markers of the speakers' internal states. Indeed, Carol Gilligan made a very important discovery about adolescent girls' development by paying close attention to the use of "I don't know" by her teenage interviewees (Gilligan & Brown, 1992).

The move from the live interview to audiotape to text progressively changes and devitalizes the interaction. Transcription, then, should try to preserve the original context as much as possible and try to capture something of the relationship in which the interview evolved. This can be done with marginal notes or commentary, and the transcription should somewhere include the notes you recorded at the conclusion of the interview.

As you listen to the interview, pay attention to yourself as an interviewer, and think about what effect you were having on the participant. You can use this time of listening as self-supervision about your interviewing stance, and think about other ways you might have better intervened (or not intervened).

At the same time (or on a second review or a review of the transcript), begin to note important themes or understandings that are emerging in relation to the question you are exploring. This will indicate what aspects of the experience you want to learn more about in the next interview. Did you get detailed enough stories? If not, you can remedy this with the next participant.

One dilemma of narrative research is how to interpret absent material. Often we expect participants to develop certain themes (perhaps ones our theories suggest are salient), and we simply don't hear about them. Later interviews give us opportunities to ask about these areas more directly, in order both to enlighten ourselves and to clarify why they may have been omitted in the earlier interviews. In a dissertation study by one of my students, the research question concerned the impact of failed love in late adolescence on adult development. To explore this issue, the student interviewed volunteers who had had a failed love experience that still affected them. He obtained rich descriptions of the love relationships in each participant's life, but after eight interviews, what was consistently missing was detailed discussion of sexuality. There were passion and romance, but no sex. What was he to make of this? In later interviews, he asked participants directly about the meanings of sexuality in the context of these love relationships, and was therefore able to write a more thorough and conceptually meaningful analysis.

The Research Relationship after the Interview

It has become popular in some research groups to do what is called "member checking," which involves asking the participants to go over transcripts of their interviews to comment on accuracy or even to review the researcher's interpretations (Lincoln & Guba, 1985). I don't do this or advise doing this unless there is some *very clear purpose* for doing so. Here is my reasoning: A participant cannot comment on the accuracy of the transcription; that can be verified only when the researcher listens to the recording along with the transcript. The researcher will only be interested in the "accuracy" of the report if the participant is construed as a witness to some outside event and if what is important to the researcher is getting "the facts" right. If what are of interest to the researcher are personal accounts and meanings, then the interview represents just one such construction. The report that the researcher creates from the interview will represent "*a* truth" rather than "*the* truth," and the researcher will assume interpretive authority for his or her understanding of the meanings of the interview material (Josselson, 2011; Chase, 1996). Where the researcher aims to discover something new, he or she may well see something that the participant does not see. In such cases, what does "disagreement" from the participant who has been "checked with" mean? Asking the participant to comment on an interpretation will produce other truths, and if these are of interest to the researcher, then reading the transcript can be a basis for a second interview that will enlarge the understandings from the first. Most participants, however, do not want to be bothered with this. They have given the interview and have now returned to their lives. The researcher, however, far from being finished with it, is just embarking on hours of review. Asking participants to review the transcripts usually leads to long delays, because they are not interested in the minutiae of the research study; all they have agreed to do is to share their experience. Of course, in collaborative action research projects, this may not be true, and a different sort of research relationship may be established; this may mean more involvement of participants in the creation of the research report. And if a researcher's aim is simply to "give voice" by re-presenting the experience of the participants, then he or she may well want to check for accuracy.

Researchers' motivations for involving participants in the analysis phase of the research project often stem from the inherent discomfort of the epistemological basis for narrative research. In a hermeneutic approach, all meanings are relative, and there is no "right" answer. The researcher takes interpretive authority (Chase, 1996) for the work. This means that the interpretations of the material are products of the researcher, who will take care in the report to document the conceptualization and to anchor it in the narrative material selected to create the argument the researcher wishes to make. The participant has no privileged point of view. The analysis is of the interview material, not of the participant (Josselson, 2011).

In the project I worked on with colleagues in which we each analyzed a single interview from our particular analytic viewpoints (Wertz et al., 2011), we asked the participant, who was a graduate student in psychology, to comment on our analyses. This led to layers of complexity. One such complexity was that the participant felt that the analysis that best represented her experience was the one done by the one of us she knew, who was actually her advisor! What we researchers agreed on was that her choice of analyses was not a reflection of who had gotten it "right." That she disputed certain interpretations some of us made did not make them incorrect. People have defenses and ways of seeing themselves that color their interpretations of the transcripts of their own interviews. We researchers, however, were not "right" either. Rather, we offered ways of viewing the narrative material that might be useful in further conceptualizing the research question. (These dilemmas are fully explored in Wertz et al., 2011, and Josselson, 2011.) For the current purposes, suffice it to say that asking for participants' input does not solve the problem of locating "truth" and creates other problems. The task of researchers in the analysis phase of the study is to document their own interpretive process and understanding in light of both the interview material and the conceptual framework they aim to apply or extend.

In most cases, the participant is not much interested in what the

researcher does with the interview material. The interview itself—
with its opportunity to talk at length, self-reflectively, with an interested listener—is reward enough. Participants are not scholars (most
of them are not, anyway) and don't care about the conceptualiza-
tions that will be addressed to scholars. They are interested in the
researcher's gratitude for their help with the project, but they usually
do not want to be burdened with other requests.

If the researcher has promised the participant a copy of the final
report—or if the participants are likely to read it on their own—
then the research relationship continues, but often in ways that the
researcher will not know about. This raises the problem that even
well-camouflaged material may still be recognizable to the persons
whose stories appear in the report. Although in each interview the
researcher has refrained from commenting on or interpreting the
participant's experience from outside the framework in which it was
offered, the research report does just this. The empathic listener has
now moved out of the stance of understanding from within the participant to talking about the participant to others. There is inevitably some betrayal in doing this—a betrayal softened perhaps by the
fact that the written report usually appears long after the interview,
so the feeling of closeness to the interviewer has lessened and the
memory of what was said has faded. Still, participants reading a
researcher's account of their experience may feel that their experience was distorted or misunderstood in some important ways. I
think it important at the close of an interview to explain something
about this phenomenon to the participant. I might say something
like this:

> I am so grateful to you for sharing your experience. I'd like to
> tell you something about what I will do with this interview.
> I am going to analyze it along with a lot of other interviews
> and try to reach some more general understanding about [the
> research topic]. Then I will selectively make use of material
> from the interviews to write about what I think I have under-
> stood. So my focus won't be on writing about *you* or about this
> experience we've just shared, but about [the research topic] and

what sense I can make of it from what I've learned from you and the other people I've interviewed.

If necessary, I can then always later remind people that I have tried to explain this.

In my decades-long concern about what it does to people to be written about in narrative research (Josselson, 1996c, 2007, 2011), I have not come across instances where people were actually harmed by participation. If identifying information is adequately disguised, then no one can identify the participants but themselves. One should write respectfully. But this doesn't mean that people won't take offense at something one has written if they recognize themselves. A participant in my longitudinal study who read a previous book I wrote about the women I have been following told me that when she read the book, she didn't like it that I said that she was "needy," but she dismissed it and decided that I had gotten this wrong. After this later interview, I checked the book, and I had not said this in relation to her or any of the other women. But this didn't mean that my participant's experience of what she thought I had said about her was any less real to her.

I have learned to bear the guilt of writing about people who have shared themselves with me. I hope that a higher good of scholarly understanding is served, and I have come to recognize, through interviewing people about the experience of being written about, that it does not harm them too painfully or irreparably. Sometimes it even makes them proud. Sometimes they think about themselves in a new and energizing way. In the end, though, our participants are usually more important to us than we are to them. We fade from their memories. But they are central to our work, and we spend hours with their interview texts; in fact, we often build our careers on what we learn from them. They stay with us throughout our lives.

CHAPTER 11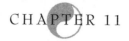

Conclusion

An in-depth interview is a special kind of conversation. The qualities of the research relationship you co-construct with your interviewees will determine the kind of sharing that will occur. Content is affected by the process. Interviewing in the ways I have detailed in this book will produce texts that reflect the nuanced complexities of life as lived by your participants. If you have listened carefully and intently, people will have told you their stories in an authentic way. If you have brought your humanity to the interviewing relationship, you will be rewarded with deeply felt accounts of experience.

I recognize that this kind of interviewing is not for everyone. It requires a toleration of uncertainty and a willingness to grapple with the complexities of a relationship's unfolding. It also requires a capacity for containing the murkiness and messiness of human feeling and experience. It is not the only way to produce knowledge, and I respect other approaches. For some of you, perhaps reading this book has persuaded you that it is not for you. For those of you committed to this approach, I hope I have given you some pointers that will assist you along the way. I hope I have also communicated my own passion for this work and indicated the joys that ensue from encountering and learning about others in this way.

The final challenge will be to return to the scholarly conversation and transform all that has enlightened you, all that has touched you, and all that you have learned into language and concepts that advance knowledge—however you think about "knowledge." This relational form of interviewing will produce texts that are suitable for narrative analysis, phenomenological analysis, discourse analysis, and grounded theory, as well as for feminist approaches, social justice orientations, or just about any other approaches you may choose for analyzing the data. But that is a subject for another book.[1]

---

[1] Again, I refer you to the Wertz et al. (2011) volume not only for the exposition, but for the excellent bibliographies for each of the approaches.

APPENDIX A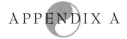

Interview Aids

Relational Space Mapping[1]

Instructions to Interviewee

"You might recall that when you were in school, you learned that the solar system looks like this." (Draw a fresh map for each interview.)

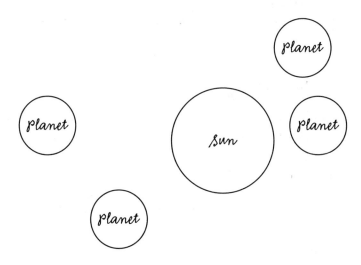

[1]See Josselson (1996b)

"I'm going to ask you to make similar diagrams, only instead of putting the sun in the middle, I want you to put yourself there. Around yourself, I'd like you to draw a circle for each person who was important to you at that time in your life, and to arrange the circles in a way that makes most sense to you. You can use as many circles as you like. By 'important,' I mean people who were in your mind, people you were thinking about. So the distance from yourself that you place each circle should reflect that person's inner importance to you, rather than whether the person was physically there or how far away he or she lived. Please label each circle with the name of the person who belongs there.

"There are two other kinds of circles you may need to draw to represent the people who mattered in your life at each time period. One is a 'dotted circle' to indicate someone who mattered a lot but wasn't there as a physical presence—for example, someone who died, or someone you only knew through reading or TV but still talked to a lot in your mind. Another kind of circle is a 'grape.' Grapes are lots of little circles to indicate a group that was important as a group, rather than individuals who mattered so much as individuals.

"I would like you to do these drawings for 5-year intervals beginning at age 5. It will be easier if you think of yourself at a particular age, rather than trying to do the years in between."

The interview following these instructions focuses on *how* each person was important.

Other Uses of This Technique

Since my initial usage of the technique described above to investigate the meanings of relationships, others have used it to understand particular kinds of relationships. For example, in Momi Beinart's (2009) study of the impact on adulthood of failed love in adolescence, he was able to see the location of each participant's loved person in the context of other relationships. Sharon Gal (2010) used these maps to investigate the relational experience of people with anorexia nervosa, and, at the end of the mapping, asked each interviewee to place the anorexia on the map as though it were a person with whom the interviewee had a relationship.

Responses to Pictures

The Thematic Apperception Test (TAT; Murray & Bellak, 1973) is a set of pictures used clinically to assess a person's internal world. It relies on the idea that stories told about these pictures reflect something about the inner fantasy life of the teller. Without accepting all the assumptions of this test, an interviewer can use any pictures to spark discussion of the participant's life. For example, Hanoch Flum (1998), studying cross-cultural experience in Ethiopian immigrants to Israel, showed them pictures from their home villages and pictures from their contemporary Israeli society (including pictures of the same people in both contexts, with varying levels of ambiguity) and asked them to tell their own stories of transition associated with the pictures.

Life Chapter Interview with or without a Timeline

In the life chapter interview technique (mentioned in Chapter 8), a participant is asked to divide his or her life into chapters, each with a title. The participant is then asked to tell about the most significant events in each chapter, particularly the high point, the low point, and a turning point (see, e.g., McAdams & Bowman, 2001). A variation of this is to ask the participant to draw a timeline of his or her life, indicating high and low points (or something else). The point of this exercise is to outline a structure that can hold the narration. One has to be careful, though, not to be too concrete about what constitutes a "high point" or "low point," because many people do not organize their life experience this way. The research needs to be sensitive to the ways in which people *do* organize their experience, and to stay within these structures.

Using Visual Representation and Technology as Interview Aids

Qualitative researchers may use a variety of visual aids to evoke or focus interview material (see Banks, 2001; Buckingham, 2009). One of my students, studying construction of bicultural identity, asked her participants to make videos of themselves holding treasured objects in their homes, and then asked them to talk about how the objects reflected the meanings of their two cultures (de Merode, 2011). Anthropologists (and others) have sometimes given people cameras to record significant scenes of their lives. The resulting pictures can be used as the basis of an interview focusing on the question to be explored.

If you are investigating the meaning of a particular event, it can be helpful to ask people to bring symbols or photos of the event. These can serve as good "launching pads" for interviews.

APPENDIX B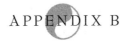

Sample Additional Questions

These questions are derived from my longitudinal study of women's identity (Josselson, 1996a)—specifically, the interview of my participants in their mid-50s. These are questions to be raised if they were appropriate to the life history of the participant but not covered in the spontaneous narration. They called attention to areas that I felt were important to explore. The little q question with which I began the interview was: "Please tell me about the last 10 years and what has been most significant for you."

"From an occupational viewpoint, what direction do you see your life taking in the future? What do you hope to be doing 10 years from now?"

"How has your marriage changed in the past 10 years? How do you fit together as a couple? How do you complement each other? In what ways do you clash?"

"How has your marriage fulfilled your needs? How has it not fulfilled your wishes? How would you like it to be different?"

"Have you had any serious marital problems? Have you seriously considered separation?"

"Which particular ages of your children's development have you found particularly enjoyable or frustrating?"

"Please tell me how you came to decide to have your first child at that particular time in your life. How did you decide on timing of subsequent children?"

"How has having children changed the person that you are? What aspects of your life (self, love relationship, career) have been enriched by motherhood, and what aspects have been diminished?"

"What has been the most difficult aspect about being a mother? What have you found hardest to adjust to? How would you like things to be different?"

"Describe the most challenging interaction or problem you've had with your children. How did you handle it?"

"How committed to your religion are you? What does your religious commitment involve?"

"Have your religious views or practices changed in the past 10 years?"

"Have your political views or preferences changed over the past 10 years?"

"How have your views about sexual morality (i.e., premarital, marital, or extramarital sex) changed over the past 10 years?"

"If you had it to do over again, what would you change about your college years?"

"What are your major hobbies or interests, and how important have they been for you?"

"What has been your philosophy over rough spots? How have you coped with stress?"

"What are your hopes, dreams, and plans for the future? How do you want your life to change in the future? In what ways do you hope to become different as a person in the future?"

"Imagine yourself at age 80 looking over your life. What would you be most satisfied to have accomplished or experienced in your life? What are the accomplishments in your life so far of which you feel most proud?"

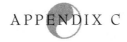

APPENDIX C

Sample Informed
Consent Form

Informed Consent Form
The Experience of Mixed-Race Youth

The title of the research should be given in simple language—so this title will appear on the consent form even if the full title of the research is "Anxiety and the Social Construction of Identity in Mixed-Race Emerging Adults.")

Thank you for responding to the recruitment letter and volunteering to participate in this study about multiracial experience.

Jane Smith, a doctoral student at Generic University, will conduct the research as part of her dissertation requirements. Millicent Jones, the dissertation chair, will supervise this study, which Generic University's Institutional Review Board (IRB) has approved.

Your participation will entail an in-depth interview, which will last approximately _____ hours. You may be asked to participate in a follow-up call to discuss your responses further and to clarify findings.

The results of this research will be published in Jane Smith's dissertation. Direct quotes from your interview may be used to clarify research conclusions. By signing this consent form, you give the researcher permission to use statements you make during the interview.

By volunteering to be interviewed, you may develop greater insight about multiracial experience and contribute to knowledge about multiraciality. No risks are anticipated with your participation in this study.

You can stop the interview at any time. You may also withdraw from this study either during or after your participation without negative consequences. Should you withdraw, your data will be eliminated from the study and destroyed.

The information you provide will be kept strictly confidential. The informed consent form will be kept separate from the interview data. The interview data will be labeled with a number code, and your name and other identifying information will be changed in the write-up of the research results to protect your identity.

If you have any questions about this study or your involvement, please ask the researcher before signing this form. If you have questions or concerns about your rights as a research participant, contact Generic University's IRB by email at xxx or by telephone at xxx. In order to ensure the ethical conduct of Generic University's researchers, the Institutional Review Board retains the right to access the signed informed consent forms and study documents.

Two copies of this informed consent form have been provided to you. Please sign both forms, indicating that you have read, understood, and agree to participate in this research. Return one to the researcher, and keep the other for your files.

Name of participant (please print) _____

Signature _____ Date _____

Contact Information

Name and address of researcher: Name and address of supervisor:

Jane Smith   *Millicent Jones*

Street address   *Street address*

Email   *Email*

Phone   *Phone*

REFERENCES

Alvesson, M., & Skoldberg, K. (2009). *Reflexive methodology: New vistas for qualitative research* (2nd ed.). Thousand Oaks, CA: Sage.

Anderson, R. (2011). Intuitive inquiry: Exploring the mirroring discourse of disease. In F. J. Wertz, K. Charmaz, L. M. McMullen, R. Josselson, R. Anderson, & E. McSpadden. *Five ways of doing qualitative analysis: Phenomenological psychology, grounded theory, discourse analysis, narrative research, and intuitive inquiry* (pp. 243–272). New York: Guilford Press.

Andrews, M. (2007). *Shaping history: Narratives of political change.* Cambridge, UK: Cambridge University Press.

Atkinson, P., Coffey, C., Delamont, S., Lofland, J., & Lofland, L. (Eds.). (2001). *Handbook of ethnography.* Thousand Oaks, CA: Sage.

Bakhtin, M. M. (1981). *The dialogic imagination.* Austin, TX: University of Texas Press.

Bakhtin, M. M. (1986). *Speech genres and other late essays.* Austin, TX: University of Texas Press.

Bamberg, M. (2006). Stories: Big or small: Why do we care? *Narrative Inquiry, 16*(1), 139–147.

Banks, M. (2001). *Visual methods in social research.* Thousand Oaks, CA: Sage.

Behar, R. (1996). *The vulnerable observer: Anthropology that breaks your heart.* Boston: Beacon Press.

Behar, R. (2003). *Translated woman: Crossing the border with Esperanza's story* (2nd ed.). Boston: Beacon Press.

Beinart, S. (2009). *The impact of primary failed love on the development of the self and future relationships: A retrospective narrative study.* Unpublished doctoral dissertation, Hebrew University, Jerusalem.

Berger, P. L., & Luckmann, T. (1966). *The social construction of reality: A treatise in the sociology of knowledge.* Garden City, NY: Anchor Books.

Bion, W. R. (1962). *Learning from experience.* London: Heinemann.

Booth, W. (1999). Doing research with lonely people. *British Journal of Learning Disabilities, 26*, 132–134.

Bourdieu, P., & Wacquant, L. J. D. (1992). *An invitation to reflexive sociology.* Chicago: University of Chicago Press.

Briggs, C. L. (1986). *Learning how to ask: A sociolinguistic appraisal of the role of the interview in social science research.* Cambridge, UK: Cambridge University Press.

Bruner, J. (1990). *Acts of meaning: Four lectures on mind and culture.* Cambridge, MA: Harvard University Press.

Buber, M. (1958). *I and Thou.* New York: Scribners.

Buckingham, D. (2009). "Creative" visual methods in media research: Possibilities, problems and proposals. *Media, Culture & Society, 31*(4), 633–652.

Cannella, G. S., & Lincoln, Y. S. (2007). Predatory vs. dialogic ethics: Constructing an illusion or ethical practice as the core of research methods. *Qualitative Inquiry, 13*(3), 315–335.

Chase, S. E. (1996). Personal vulnerability and interpretive authority in narrative research. In R. Josselson (Ed.), *Ethics and process in the narrative study of lives* (pp. 45–59). Thousand Oaks, CA: Sage.

Clandinin, D. J., & Connelly, F. M. (2000). *Narrative inquiry: Experience and story in qualitative research.* San Francisco: Jossey-Bass.

Clarke, S., & Hoggett, P. (Eds.). (2009). *Researching beneath the surface: Psycho-social research methods in practice.* London: Karnac Books.

Cohen, S. K. (2005). *Child survivors of the Holocaust in Israel: Finding their voice: Social dynamics and post-war experiences.* Brighton, UK: Sussex Academic Press.

Cohler, B. (1982). Personal narratives and the life course. In P. B. Baltes & O. G. Brim, Jr. (Eds.), *Life-span development and behavior* (Vol. 4, pp. 205–241). New York: Academic Press.

Creswell, J. W. (2012). *Qualitative inquiry and research design: Choosing among five approaches.* Thousand Oaks, CA: Sage.

de Merode, J. (2011). *Two halves make a whole: Evidence of integration in bicultural adults' chosen visual symbols of self-identity.* Unpublished doctoral dissertation, Fielding Graduate University.

Denzin, N. K., & Lincoln, Y. S. (Eds.). (2011). *The Sage handbook of qualitative research* (4th ed.). Thousand Oaks, CA: Sage.

Eakin, P. J. (2008). *Living autobiographically: How we create identity in narrative.* Ithaca, NY: Cornell University Press.

Ellenbogen, G. C. (Ed.). (1987). *Oral sadism and the vegetarian personality.* New York: Brunner/Mazel.

Ellis, C. (2009). *Revision: Autoethnographic reflections on life and work.* Walnut Creek, CA: Left Coast Press.

Fine, M. (1994). Working the hyphens: Reinventing self and other in qualitative research. In N. K. Denzin & Y. S. Lincoln (Eds.), *Handbook of qualitative research* (pp. 70–82). Thousand Oaks, CA: Sage.

Fine, M., Weis, L., Wong, L. M., & Weseen, S. (2000). For whom? Qualitative research, representations, and social responsibilities. In N. Denzin & Y. Lincoln (Eds.), *The handbook of qualitative research* (2nd ed., pp. 107–131). Thousand Oaks, CA: Sage.

Flum, H. (1998). Embedded identity: The case of young high-achieving Ethiopian Jewish immigrants in Israel. *Journal of Youth Studies, 1*(2), 143–161.

Forrester, A. M. (2002). *The telling of the telling: A narrative exploration of adolescent girls' process of disclosure of sexual abuse.* Unpublished doctoral dissertation, Fielding Graduate University.

Fosshage, J. L. (1995). Countertransference as the analyst's experience of the analysand: Influence of listening perspectives. *Psychoanalytic Psychology, 12*(3), 375.

Fulford, R. (1999). *The triumph of narrative: Storytelling in the age of mass culture.* New York: Broadway Books.

Gadamer, H.-G. (1975). *Truth and method* (G. Barden & J. Cumming, Eds. & Trans.). New York: Seabury Press.

Gal, S. (2010). *The relational patterns, dimensions and meanings of anorexia nervosa.* Unpublished doctoral dissertation, Hebrew University, Jerusalem.

Geertz, C. (1988). *Works and lives: The anthropologist as author.* Stanford, CA: Stanford University Press.

Gergen, K. J. (1994). *Realities and relationships: Soundings in social construction.* Cambridge, MA: Harvard University Press.

Gergen, K. J. (2009). *Relational being: Beyond self and community.* New York: Oxford University Press.

Gilbert, K. R. (Ed.). (2001). *The emotional nature of qualitative research.* Boca Raton, FL: CRC Press.

Gilligan, C., & Brown, L. M. (1992). *Meeting at the crossroads.* Cambridge, MA: Harvard University Press.

Goldberg, S. G. (2007). *The social construction of bipolar disorder: The interre-

lationship between societal and individual meanings. Unpublished doctoral dissertation, Fielding Graduate University.

Granek, L. (2011). Putting ourselves on the line: Intersubjectivity and social responsibility in qualitative research. *International Journal of Qualitative Studies in Education.* Retrieved from *www.tandfonline.com/doi/abs/10.1080/09518398.2011.614645#preview*

Granek, L. (2012). The bits on the cutting room floor: Erasures and denials within the qualitative research trajectory. *Psychotherapy and Social Sciences, 14*(2).

Greenspan, H. (2010). *On listening to Holocaust survivors: Beyond testimony* (2nd ed.). St. Paul, MN: Paragon House.

Gregg, G. S. (2006). The raw and the bland: A structural model of narrative identity. In D. P. McAdams, R. Josselson, & A. Lieblich (Eds.), *Identity and story: Creating self in narrative* (pp. 63–87). Washington, DC: American Psychological Association.

Gubrium, J. F., & Holstein, J. A. (2002). *Handbook of interview research: Context and method.* Thousand Oaks, CA: Sage.

Hollway, W., & Jefferson, T. (2000). *Doing qualitative research differently: Free association, narrative and the interview method.* Thousand Oaks, CA: Sage.

Janesick, V. J. (2010). *Oral history for the qualitative researcher.* New York: Guilford Press.

Janesick, V. J. (2011). *"Stretching" exercises for qualitative researchers* (3rd ed.). Thousand Oaks, CA: Sage.

Josselson, R. (1996a). *Revising herself: The story of women's identity from college to midlife.* New York: Oxford University Press.

Josselson, R. (1996b). *The space between us: Exploring the dimensions of human relationships.* Thousand Oaks, CA: Sage.

Josselson, R. (1996c). On writing other people's lives. In R. Josselson (Ed.), *Ethics and process in the narrative study of lives* (pp. 60–71). Thousand Oaks, CA: Sage.

Josselson, R. (2004). The hermeneutics of faith and the hermeneutics of suspicion. *Narrative Inquiry, 14*(1), 1–28.

Josselson, R. (2007). The ethical attitude in narrative research: Principles and practicalities. In D. J. Clandinin (Ed.), *Handbook of narrative inquiry* (pp. 537–567). Thousand Oaks, CA: Sage.

Josselson, R. (2011). "Bet you think this song is about you": Whose narrative is it in narrative research? *Narrative Works, 1*(1). Retrieved from *http://journals.hil.unb.ca/index.php/NW/article/view/18472*

Kerem, E., Fishman, N., & Josselson, R. (2001). The experience of empathy in everyday relationships: Cognitive and affective elements. *Journal of Social and Personal Relationships, 18*(5), 709–729.

Kitzinger, C., & Wilkinson, S. (1996). Theorizing representing the other. In S. Wilkinson & C. Kitzinger (Eds.), *Representing the other: A feminism and psychology reader* (pp. 1–32). London: Sage.

Krumer-Nevo, M. (2002). The arena of othering: A narrative study with women living in poverty and social marginality. *Qualitative Social Work, 1*(3), 303–318.

Krumer-Nevo , M., & Sidi, M. (2012). Writing against othering. *Qualitative Inquiry, 18*, 299–309.

Kvale, S. (1996). *InterViews: An introduction to qualitative research interviewing.* Thousand Oaks, CA: Sage.

Kvale, S., & Brinkmann, S. (2009). *InterViews: Learning the craft of qualitative research interviewing* (2nd ed.). Thousand Oaks, CA: Sage.

Labov, W., & Waletzky, J. (1967). Narrative analysis: Oral versions of personal experience. In J. Helm (Ed.), *Essays on the verbal and visual arts: Proceedings of the 196th Annual Spring Meeting of the American Ethnological Society* (pp. 12–44). Seattle: University of Washington Press.

Lieblich, A. (1996). Some unforeseen outcomes of conducting narrative research with people of one's own culture. In R. Josselson (Ed.), *Ethics and process in the narrative study of lives* (pp. 172–186). Thousand Oaks, CA: Sage.

Lieblich, A., Tuval-Mashiach, R., & Zilber, T. (1998). *Narrative research: Reading, analysis, and interpretation.* Thousand Oaks, CA: Sage.

Lincoln, Y. S. (2005). Institutional review boards and methodological conservatism: The challenge to and from phenomenological paradigms. In N. K. Denzin & Y. S. Lincoln (Eds.), *Handbook of qualitative research* (3rd ed., pp. 165–181). Thousand Oaks, CA: Sage.

Lincoln, Y. S., & Guba, E. G. (1985). *Naturalistic inquiry.* Thousand Oaks, CA: Sage.

Linde, C. (1993). *Life stories: The creation of coherence.* New York: Oxford University Press.

Linde, C. (2008). *Working the past: Narrative and institutional memory.* New York: Oxford University Press.

Lomsky-Fedder, E. (1996). A woman studies war: Stranger in a man's world. In R. Josselson (Ed.), *Ethics and process in the narrative study of lives* (pp. 232–244). Thousand Oaks, CA: Sage.

Lyotard, J.-F. (1984). *The postmodern condition: A report on knowledge* (G. Bennington & B. Massumi, Trans.). Minneapolis: University of Minnesota Press.

MacIntyre, A. (2007). *After virtue: A study in moral theory* (3rd ed.). Notre Dame, IN: University of Notre Dame Press.

McAdams, D. P., & Bowman, P. J. (2001). Narrating life's turning points: Redemption and contamination. In D. P. McAdams, R. Josselson, & A. Lieblich (Eds.), *Turns in the road: Narrative studies of lives in transition* (pp. 3–34). Washington, DC: American Psychological Association.

McAdams, D. P., Josselson, R., & Lieblich, A. (Eds.). (2001). *Turns in the road: Narrative studies of lives in transition*. Washington, DC: American Psychological Association.

McAdams, D. P., Josselson, R., & Lieblich, A. (Eds.). (2006). *Identity and story: Creating self in narrative*. Washington, DC: American Psychological Association.

Messer, S. B., Sass, L. A., & Woolfolk, R. L. (Eds.). (1988). *Hermeneutics and psychological theory: Interpretive perspectives on personality, psychotherapy, and psychopathology*. New Brunswick, NJ: Rutgers University Press.

Miller, M. (1996). Ethics and understanding through interrelationship: I and thou in dialogue. In R. Josselson (Ed.), *Ethics and process in the narrative study of lives* (pp. 129–150). Thousand Oaks, CA: Sage.

Mishler, E. G. (1986). *Research interviewing: Context and narrative*. Cambridge, MA: Harvard University Press.

Murray, H. A., & Bellak, L. (1973). *Thematic Apperception Test*. New York: Psychological Corporation.

Nasim, R. (2007). Ongoing relationships: Recounting a lost parent's life as a means to remember. In R. Josselson, A. Lieblich, & D. P. McAdams (Eds.), *The meaning of others: Narrative studies of relationships* (pp. 255–280). Washington, DC: American Psychological Association.

Orange, D. M. (2011). *The suffering stranger: Hermeneutics for everyday clinical practice*. New York: Routledge.

Ouellette, S. (2003). Painting lessons. In R. Josselson, A. Lieblich, & D. McAdams (Eds.), *Up close and personal: The teaching and learning of narrative research* (pp. 13–28). Washington, DC: APA Books.

Patai, D. (1991). U.S. academics and third-world women: Is ethical research possible? In S. Gluck & D. Patai (Eds.), *Women's words: The feminist practice of oral history* (pp. 137–153). New York: Routledge.

Pennebaker, J. W., & Chung, C. K. (2007). Expressive writing, emotional upheavals, and health. *Foundations of Health Psychology*, 263–284.

Pennebaker, J. W., & Seagal, J. D. (1999). Forming a story: The health benefits of narrative. *Journal of Clinical Psychology, 55*(10), 1243–1254.

Polkinghorne, D. E. (1988). *Narrative knowing and the human sciences*. Albany: State University of New York Press.

Potter, J., & Wetherell, M. (1987). *Discourse and social psychology: Beyond attitudes and behaviour*. Thousand Oaks, CA: Sage.

Ricoeur, P. (1981). *Hermeneutics and the human sciences* (J. B. Thompson, Ed. & Trans.). Cambridge, UK: Cambridge University Press.

Rogers, A., Holland, J., Casey, M. E., Nakkula, V., Ekert, J., & Sheinberg, N. (1999). An interpretive poetics of languages of the unsayable. In R. Josselson & A. Lieblich (Eds.), *The narrative study of lives: Vol. 6. Making meaning of narratives* (pp. 77–106). Thousand Oaks, CA: Sage.

Rogers, A. G. (2007). The unsayable, Lacanian psychoanalysis, and the art of narrative intervieweing. In J. D. Clandinin (Ed.), *Handbook of narrative inquiry* (pp. 99–119). Thousand Oaks, CA: Sage.

Rosenwald, G. (1996). Making whole: Method and ethics in mainstream and narrative psychology. In R. Josselson (Ed.), *Ethics and process in the narrative study of lives* (pp. 245–274). Thousand Oaks, CA: Sage.

Roulston, K. J. (2010). *Reflective interviewing: A guide to theory and practice*. Thousand Oaks, CA: Sage.

Sands, R. G., & Krumer-Nevo, M. (2006). Interview shocks and shock-waves. *Qualitative Inquiry, 12*(5), 950–971.

Sarbin, T. R. (1986). *Narrative psychology: The storied nature of human conduct*. New York: Praeger.

Sayer, A. (1992). *Method in social science: A realist approach*. New York: Routledge.

Seidman, I. (2006). *Interviewing as qualitative research: A guide for researchers in education and the social sciences* (3rd ed.). New York: Teachers College Press.

Simon, R. (2012). Men's views of work–life balance: A phenomenological study. *Dissertation Abstracts International, 72*(10), 6399B.

Spence, D. P. (1984). *Narrative truth and historical truth: Meaning and interpretation in psychoanalysis*. New York: Norton.

Stolorow, R., Atwood, G., & Orange, D. (2002). *Worlds of experience: Interweaving philosophical and clinical dimensions in psychoanalysis*. New York: Basic Books.

Weiss, R. S. (1994). *Learning from strangers: The art and method of qualitative interview studies*. New York: Free Press.

Wertz, F. J., Charmaz, K., McMullen, L. M., Josselson, R., Anderson, R., & McSpadden, E. (2011). *Five ways of doing qualitative analysis: Phenomenological psychology, grounded theory, discourse analysis, narrative research, and intuitive inquiry.* New York: Guilford Press.

Willig, C. (2003). Discourse analysis. In J. A. Smith (Ed.), *Qualitative psychology: A practical guide to research methods* (pp. 159–183). Thousand Oaks, CA: Sage.

Index

ABOUT THE AUTHOR

Ruthellen Josselson, PhD, is Professor of Clinical Psychology at Fielding Graduate University. She was formerly Professor at The Hebrew University of Jerusalem, Visiting Professor at Harvard University School of Education, and Visiting Fellow at Cambridge University. Dr. Josselson is a cofounder of the Society for Qualitative Inquiry in Psychology; coeditor of 11 volumes of *The Narrative Study of Lives,* a series dedicated to publishing qualitative research; coauthor of *Five Ways of Doing Qualitative Analysis;* and author of many journal articles and book chapters that explore the theory and practice of qualitative inquiry. She has conducted workshops on interviewing skills for qualitative inquiry in the United States, France, Norway, Finland, Israel, and the United Kingdom. Based on interviews she has conducted over 35 years, she has written two books exploring women's identity longitudinally (*Finding Herself* and *Revising Herself*) and three other books (*The Space Between Us, Best Friends,* and *Playing Pygmalion*). Dr. Josselson is a recipient of the American Psychological Association's Henry A. Murray Award and Theodore R. Sarbin Award as well as a Fulbright Fellowship.